Multidetector-Row Computed Tomography
Scanning and Contrast Protocols

G. Marchal • **T. J. Vogl** • **J. P. Heiken** • **G. D. Rubin** (Eds)

Multidetector-Row Computed Tomography

Scanning and Contrast Protocols

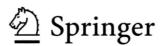

Springer

Guy Marchal
Department of Radiology
University Hospitals Leuven
Leuven, Belgium

Thomas J. Vogl
Department of Radiology
University of Frankfurt
Frankfurt am Main, Germany

Jay P. Heiken
Mallinckrodt Institute of Radiology
Washington University School of Medicine
St. Louis, USA

Geoffrey D. Rubin
Department of Radiology
Stanford University School of Medicine
Stanford, USA

ISBN 88-470-0305-9 Springer Milan Berlin Heidelberg New York

Library of Congress Control Number: 2005921141

Springer is a part of Springer Science+Business Media
springeronline.com
© Springer-Verlag Italia 2005
Printed in Italy

Cover design: Simona Colombo, Milan
Typesetting: Compostudio, Cernusco s/N (Milan)
Printing and binding: Arti Grafiche Nidasio, Assago (Milan)

Preface

The discovery of X-rays by Konrad Roentgen is one of the major milestones in the history of modern medicine, allowing for the first time a noninvasive look inside the patient. Two-dimensional X-ray images remained the basis of clinical radiology until the early 1970s when computerized cross-sectional imaging with computed tomography (CT) and ultrasound became routinely available.

Cross-sectional imaging did indeed dramatically change our knowledge of the incidence and the evolution of many diseases. It rapidly became the basic clinical tool for diagnosis and follow-up and had a fundamental impact on medicine.

A second revolution started in the early 1980s with the clinical introduction of magnetic resonance imaging (MRI). At that time the excitement among radiologists was such that many believed MRI would rapidly replace CT and even ultrasound for most of the diagnostic work. MRI with its fantastic soft-tissue contrast, its multiplanar imaging capability, the potential of tissue- or organ-specific contrast agents, and last but not least the absence of ionizing radiation seemed a technique difficult to beat. On top of this, the evolution of MR technology was so fast, that most limitations which characterized the early MR systems were rapidly overcome, and this evolution is still ongoing. CT seemed completely outperformed and outdated even though volumetric acquisition with spiral technology was already widely available at that time.

Even the introduction of the first dual-slice spiral scanner did not receive too much attention. On the contrary, most radiology departments invested massively in the acquisition of MR magnets and many changed their name from "radiology" to "imaging" departments.

However, things started to change with the introduction of the first four-slice spiral CT scanners in 1998. Multidetector-row technology caused a worldwide revival of CT. The reason for this revival resides in the amazing technical advancements in the hardware and software offered by these new devices.

Today, the latest multidetector-row CT (MDCT) scanners offer the possibility to perform volumetric submillimetric isotropic imaging of large body areas in only a few seconds. These data can be reviewed and even directly reconstructed in any arbitrary plane.

If needed, the acquisitions can be gated to freeze the cardiac motion, and if multiphase images are reconstructed, functional information can be extracted from the time sequences. As a result many of the features which were considered typical advantages of MRI are today also available on a standard MDCT scanner.

However, CT remains X-ray based and therefore unfortunately still has a number of weak points compared to MRI, including the lower soft-tissue contrast and the use of ionizing radiation. On the other hand, CT has the advantage of being less complicated to perform and to interpret.

Still, to take full advantage of modern MDCT technology, radiologists have to reconsider their acquisition protocols, particularly regarding timing and the administration of contrast media.

It is obvious that once the total acquisition time of an examination is reduced to only a few seconds, one has to take into account the normal and/or abnormal vascular physiology of the patient.

Acquisition parameters, injection regimes, timing, and contrast concentrations have to be individually optimized. Without a very careful approach many of the benefits of a fast CT scan are often lost and the images become suboptimal or even unreadable.

The workflow of CT also has to be reengineered. Currently, patient preparation and data acquisition represent only a minor part of the total workflow. Efficient data transfer, archiving, three-dimensional processing, and image interpretation become increasingly demanding on hard- and software because of the massive amounts of data produced.

The goal of the present volume is to provide practical answers to the questions most often raised. The authors sought to come up with state-of-the-art protocols and solutions for the different generations of MDCT scanners currently available on the market and in doing so, they hope that this book will help the readers to get the most out of their equipment.

January 2005

Guy Marchal
Dept. of Radiology
Leuven, Belgium

Contents

SECTION IV – Future Prospects in MDCT Imaging

Contributors

E. Freddy Avni
Department of Radiology
Erasme Hospital
Brussels, Belgium

Kyongtae T. Bae
Mallinckrodt Institute of Radiology
Washington University School
of Medicine
St. Louis, USA

Christoph R. Becker
Department of Clinical Radiology
University Hospital Grosshadern
Munich, Germany

Linda Bertoletti
Department of Radiological Sciences
Policlinico Umberto I
Rome, Italy

Carlo Catalano
Department of Radiological Sciences
Policlinico Umberto I
Rome, Italy

Mario Cavacece
Department of Radiological Sciences
Policlinico Umberto I
Rome, Italy

Claus D. Claussen
Department of Diagnostic Radiology
Eberhard-Karls University Tuebingen
Tuebingen, Germany

Arielle Crombé-Ternamian
Service de Radiologie Digestive
Hôpital Edouard Herriot
Lyon, France

Johan de Mey
Radiology and Medical Imaging
Brussels, Belgium

Steven Dymarkowski
Radiological, Cardiovascular and
Abdominal Imaging
University Hospital Gasthuisberg
Leuven, Belgium

Dominik Fleischmann
Department of Radiology
Stanford University Medical Center
Stanford, USA

Francesco Fraioli
Department of Radiological Sciences
Policlinico Umberto I
Rome, Italy

Renate M. Hammerstingl
Department of Diagnostic and
Interventional Radiology
Johann Wolfgang Goethe University
Frankfurt am Main, Germany

Jay P. Heiken
Mallinckrodt Institute of Radiology
Washington University School
of Medicine
St. Louis, USA

Christopher Herzog
Department of Radiology
University of Frankfurt
Frankfurt am Main, Germany

Martin Heuschmid
Department of Diagnostic Radiology
Eberhard-Karls University Tuebingen
Tuebingen, Germany

Andreas F. Kopp
Department of Diagnostic Radiology
Eberhard-Karls University Tuebingen
Tuebingen, Germany

Axel Küttner
Department of Diagnostic Radiology
Eberhard-Karls University Tuebingen
Tuebingen, Germany

Kenneth A. Miles
Brighton & Sussex Medical School
University of Brighton
Brighton, UK

Alfonso Marchianò
Istituto Nazionale dei Tumori
Milan, Italy

Alessandro Napoli
Department of Radiological Sciences
Policlinico Umberto I
Rome, Italy

Piergiorgio Nardis
Department of Radiological Sciences
Policlinico Umberto I
Rome, Italy

Paul Parizel
Department of Radiology
University of Antwerp
Edegem, Belgium

Roberto Passariello
Department of Radiological Sciences
Policlinico Umberto I
Rome, Italy

Frank Pilleul
Service de Radiologie Digestive
Hôpital Edouard Herriot
Lyon, France

Mathias Prokop
Department of Radiology
University Medical Center Utrecht
Utrecht, The Netherlands

Geoffrey D. Rubin
Department of Radiology
Stanford University School of Medicine
Stanford, USA

Stephen Schröder
Department of Diagnostic Radiology
Eberhard-Karls University Tuebingen
Tuebingen, Germany

Alberto Spinazzi
Bracco Diagnostics Inc.
Princeton, USA

Pierre-Jean Valette
Department of Digestive Radiology
Hôpital Edouard Herriot
Lyon, France

Bernard E. Van Beers
Diagnostic Radiology Unit
Saint-Luc University Hospital
Brussels, Belgium

Koenraad Verstraete
Department of Radiology
Ghent University Hospital
Ghent, Belgium

Thomas J. Vogl
Department of Radiology
University of Frankfurt
Frankfurt am Main, Germany

SECTION I

Principles and Challenges of MDCT

I

Introduction

E. Freddy Avni

Multidetector row computed tomography (MDCT) has modified the imaging approach for the assessment of many diseases. The technique enables the acquisition of a volume of data, rather than slices. The most recent clinical developments involving this technique include the screening of colorectal polyps, the detection of lung nodules, the screening for cardiac and coronary artery diseases, and the easy three-dimensional rendering of various vessels in any part of the body.

Advantages of the technique include the rapid acquisition and three-dimensional rendering of images even of the pulsating heart or vessels. The spatial resolution is improving and so is the diagnostic confidence. Due to the faster acquisition time, we are moving towards automated procedures of acquisition and image reading.

However, there are several challenges that radiology departments face in the use of this rapidly evolving technique. These challenges include (among others).

- Management of the workload of a CT suite; today it takes more time to position patients than to acquire the images. The organization of the day-to-day work must be optimized.
- The number of images to be read by the radiologist has dramatically increased. The time necessary for their interpretation is also increasing. In the very near future, automatic three-dimensional rendering of the raw data will simplify this.
- The rapid translation of the table may increase the number of motion artifacts. Various methods have already been developed to reduce motion artifacts.
- The rate of injection and volume of contrast needed for the examinations have to be adapted. High-concentration contrast media are now preferable.

Of utmost importance is the control of the radiation delivered during a MDCT examination, both in children and in adults. The manufacturers are progressively introducing methods that will allow the radiation dose to be reduced. For instance, attenuation-based online modulation of the tube current in order to reduce the milliampere settings has now become commercially available and this permits a dose reduction without loss of image quality.

Important questions that need to be answered soon concern the evaluation of the clinical impact of systematic screenings that all radiologists tend to perform (i.e., for pulmonary nodules). Are we doing better? Are we improving the medical care and outcome?

Finally, other techniques are also able to provide the same or similar clinical information; comparisons are necessary in order to choose the best technique and to reduce cost and optimize patient management.

Suggested Reading

Fleischmann D (2003) Use of high-concentration contrast media in multiple-detector-row CT: principles and rationale. Eur Radiol 13 [Suppl 5]:M14-M20

Akbar SA, Mortele KJ, Baeyens K et al (2004) Multidetector CT urography: techniques, clinical applications, and pitfalls. Semin Ultrasound CT MR 25:41-54

Kelly DM, Hasegawa I, Borders R et al (2004) High-resolution CT using MDCT: comparison of degree of motion artifact between volumetric and axial methods. AJR Am J Roentgenol 182:757-759

Roos JE, Desbiolles LM, Weishaupt D et al (2004) Multidetector row CT: effect of iodine dose reduction on hepatic and vascular enhancement. Rofo Fortschr Geb Rontgenstr Neuen Bildgeb Verfahr 176:556-563

Schoellnast H, Tillich M, Deutschmann HA et al (2004) Improvement of parenchymal and vascular enhancement using saline flush and power injection for multiple-detector-row abdominal CT. Eur Radiol 14:659-664

Ferencik M, Moselewski F, Ropers D et al (2003) Quantitative parameters of image quality in multidetector spiral computed tomographic coronary imaging with submillimeter collimation. Am J Cardiol 92:1257-1262

Herzog C, Britten M, Balzer JO et al (2004) Multidetector-row cardiac CT: diagnostic value of calcium scoring and CT coronary angiography in patients with symptomatic, but atypical, chest pain. Eur Radiol 14:169-177

Achenbach S, Moselewski F, Ropers D et al (2004) Detection of calcified and noncalcified coronary atherosclerotic plaque by contrast-enhanced, submillimeter multidetector spiral computed tomography: a segment-based comparison with intravascular ultrasound. Circulation 109:14-17

Hoffmann MH, Shi H, Schmid FT et al (2004) Noninvasive coronary imaging with MDCT in comparison to invasive conventional coronary angiography: a fast-developing technology. AJR Am J Roentgenol 182:601-608

Fleischmann D (2003) MDCT of renal and mesenteric vessels. Eur Radiol 13 [Suppl 5]:M94-M101

Nasir K, Budoff MJ, Post WS et al (2003) Electron beam CT versus helical CT scans for assessing coronary calcification: current utility and future directions. Am Heart J 146:969-977

Macari M, Bini EJ, Jacobs SL et al (2004) Colorectal polyps and cancers in asymptomatic average-risk patients: evaluation with CT colonography. Radiology 230:629-636

Morrin MM, Kruskal JB, Farrell RJ et al (1999) Endoluminal CT colonography after an incomplete endoscopic colonoscopy. AJR Am J Roentgenol 172:913-918

Cody DD, Moxley DM, Krugh KT et al (2004) Strategies for formulating appropriate MDCT techniques when imaging the chest, abdomen, and pelvis in pediatric patients. AJR Am J Roentgenol 182:849-859

Grude M, Juergens KU, Wichter T et al (2003) Evaluation of global left ventricular myocardial function with electrocardiogram-gated multidetector computed tomography: comparison with magnetic resonance imaging. Invest Radiol 38:653-661

I.1

MDCT: Technical Principles and Future Trends

Mathias Prokop

Introduction

Multidetector-row computed tomography (MDCT), also known as multislice, multidetector CT, or multisection CT, is the latest breakthrough in CT technology. It has transformed CT from a transaxial cross-sectional technique into a truly three-dimensional imaging modality. While dual-slice spiral scanning has been available since 1992, the first four-slice units were introduced in 1998 [1, 2]. Systems with 6-, 8-, 10-, and 16-detector arrays have become available over the past few years, and scanners with 32-, 40-, and 64-detector rows will be introduced in 2004. MDCT has been more rapidly accepted in the radiological community than single-slice spiral CT, with exponential growth in the use of these scanners in clinical practice worldwide, from 10 scanners in 1998 to 100 in 1999, to 1,000 in 2000, and over 5,000 by 2002.

Advantages of MDCT

The main problem with spiral CT scanning is the inverse relationship between scan length and spatial resolution along the patient axis (z-axis resolution). Thus, a volumetric acquisition with high spatial resolution in all spatial directions can only cover small areas during one breath hold.

The solution to this problem is to acquire multiple simultaneous slices and use a higher speed of rotation. As a result, a four-detector row scanner with 0.5-s rotation, for example, has a performance that is up to eight times greater than a conventional 1-s single-slice scanner. This allows high spatial resolution to be achieved over a long scan range. However, scan duration cannot be reduced with four-slice systems with this approach. If the scan duration is decreased with four-slice systems, then either the scan length or z-axis resolution must be reduced. With 8- to 16-detector rows, however, re-duced scan durations can be achieved despite high z-axis resolution.

The advantages of MDCT compared with single-detector-row CT are summarized in Table 1. With faster scans, a smaller than usual quantity of contrast medium can be used for indications in which only opacification of vascular structures is important [e.g., CT angiography (CTA)] [3]. Movement artifacts are less problematic with MDCT, in particular with 8- to 16-slice scanners. Longer scan ranges are the prerequisite for high-resolution CT (HRCT) of the entire chest or for peripheral CTA (Fig. 1). The main breakthrough of MDCT has been in the area of thinner sections, which makes it possible to acquire a (near) isotropic data vol-

Table 1. Advantages of MDCT

Shorter scan duration
Reduced movement artifacts:
• Children
• Trauma patients
• Acutely ill or dyspneic patients
• Multiplanar reformations
Improved contrast-enhanced scans:
• Well-defined phase of contrast enhancement
• Reduced contrast volume for CTA
• More-homogeneous enhancement
Longer scan ranges
CTA
• Aorta and peripheral run-off
• Thoraco-abdominal aorta
• Carotids from arch to intracerebral circulation
Trauma
• Full spine examinations
Thinner sections
Near-isotropic imaging (any application):
• Arbitrary imaging planes
• Multiplanar reformations
• Three-dimensional rendering

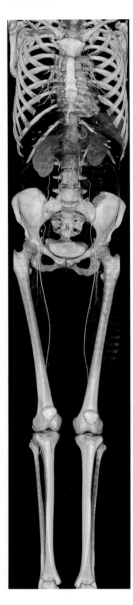

Fig. 1. CTA of the whole aorta and peripheral run-off vessels in a patient with Leriche syndrome (16×0.75 mm), reconstructed at 0.7-mm intervals, resulted in over 2,000 axial images

ume [4, 5]. As a consequence, arbitrary cross-sectional planes [multiplanar reformations (MPR)] can be reconstructed from the data volume and excellent three-dimensional displays become possible.

Disadvantages of MDCT

The advantages of MDCT come with the problem of a markedly increased *data load*. More than 1,000 images can be produced (Fig. 1), particularly with near-isotropic volume acquisition techniques [6]. While such a volumetric acquisition is used less frequently with most 4-slice scanners, it is a standard technique for 16-slice scanners. The number of images depends on the scan range, the reconstruction interval, and the number of series to be reconstructed. The large data load means that new ways of viewing, processing, archiving, and demonstrating images are necessary, and more time is needed to analyze the data than with single-slice spiral CT.

Image noise grows as the section collimation is reduced. To keep the noise low, either the radiation dose needs to be raised or thicker sections have to be reconstructed. In addition, the *geometric efficiency* of the detectors deteriorates with very thin collimation. This effect is most prominent for four-slice scanners at 0.5–0.625-mm collimation and accounts for an increase in dose requirements (volume CT dose index, $CTDI_{vol}$) by a factor of more than 2. Even at 1–1.25-mm collimation, the CT dose index is still 30%–50% larger than at a 5-mm collimation or a single-slice scanner under otherwise identical conditions [7]. The increase in dose requirements varies between scanner manufacturers and depends on the implementation of beam collimation and image interpolation algorithms. With 8- and 16-row scanners there is a substantial improvement in dose efficiency. The increase in $CTDI_{vol}$ in 16-slice units is well below 10% and can therefore be neglected in clinical practice.

Radiation dose is substantially increased in MDCT if the same milliampere settings are used as in single-slice scanning [8], but careful choice of scanning parameters can avoid this problem. Increased radiation dose per milliampere compared with single-slice CT can be due to differences in scanner geometry (such as a reduced tube-detector distance in GE units), pre-filtering, or the display of effective milliampere settings instead of the real milliampere settings on the user interface (on Philips and Siemens units). The latter approach is based on the concept that the effective milliampere (mA/pitch) is by definition independent of the pitch factor and therefore serves as a better indicator of the patient dose [1]. However, if a user implements an MDCT protocol with identical settings as on a single-slice scanner by the same manufacturer, he will actually increase the patient dose (by the pitch factor he had used on his single-slice unit) because the milliampere indicated on the MDCT interface actually represents the effective milliampere.

For these reasons, it is advisable to design scanning protocols that are not based on previous milliampere settings but on actual dose values as indicated by the $CTDI_{vol}$, which are now displayed on the user interface of all MDCT scanners (in some countries this option is only made available upon request by the customer). As a consequence of prudent selection of parameters, an increased radiation dose with MDCT is only needed if thin-section images of high quality are re-

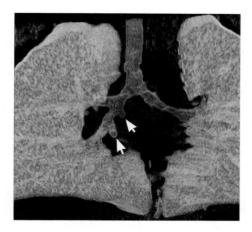

Fig. 2. Low-dose scan (CTDI$_{vol}$ <3 mGy) in a non-anesthetized child using 4×1-mm collimation. Two accessory bronchial buds (*arrows*) are visible on the volume-rendered image

quired. If scanning parameters are chosen carefully, MDCT requires a lower radiation dose than conventional CT or a similar dose to spiral CT with a pitch of 2. It is therefore essential to optimize scan protocols. Doses should be as low as possible for scans of children (Fig. 2) and patients of small stature [7].

A low kVp setting can be used to increase the CT attenuation of iodinated contrast material and thus improve the contrast of perfused structures [9]. The resulting gain in signal-to-noise ratio can be used to save dose while maintaining a reasonably good image quality. The technique works best in the chest (e.g., CTA of pulmonary embolism [10]) but can also be used in the head, neck, or in the abdomen of slim patients (Fig. 3). It is particularly useful for the examination of children. In regions with increased X-ray attenuation, such as the abdomen or in obese patients, the attenuation becomes disproportionately high and a low kVp technique should not be applied.

Detector Types

The current MDCT scanners acquire 2, 4, 6, 8, 10, or 16 simultaneous sections. Scanners with 32–, 40–, or 64– detector rows are now also available. The actual number of detector rows is usually much larger than the active number of detector rows in order to achieve more than one collimation setting. This is achieved by collimating and adding together the signals of neighboring detector rows.

There are three types of detector arrays: matrix detectors, which consist of parallel rows of equal thickness, hybrid detectors with smaller detector rows in the center, and adaptive array detectors that consist of detector rows with varying thickness (Fig. 4). While GE uses a matrix detector for their four- and eight-slice systems, Philips and Siemens have opted for an adaptive array configuration for their four-slice systems (Siemens also for their six-slice system). Hybrid detectors have

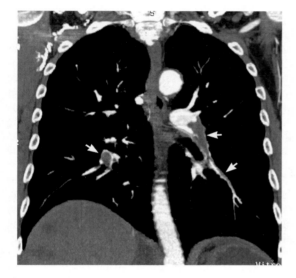

Fig. 3. Low-dose CTA using 80 kVp (CTDI$_{vol}$ >2.5 mGy) on a 4-slice scanner (4×1-mm collimation) demostrates multiple pulmonary emboli, some of which are already partially resorbed

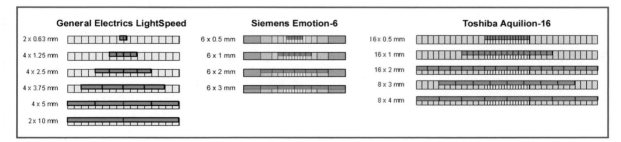

Fig. 4. Examples of a 4-slice matrix detector (GE LightSpeed), a 6-slice adaptive array detector (Siemens Emotion-6), and a 16-slice hybrid detector (Toshiba Aquilion-16)

been adopted by Toshiba for their 4- to 16-slice systems, but are also used in all 10- to 16-row scanners from other manufacturers.

The coming generation of 32- to 64-slice scanners is based on matrix geometry (GE, Toshiba) or hybrid geometry (Philips, Siemens). Since many of these systems are still under development, specifications may be changed before final release. GE will provide a scanner with 64×0.625-mm collimation that can also acquire data with 32×1.25-mm collimation. Philips uses a hybrid configuration that provides 40×0.625-mm and 32×1.25-mm collimation for their Brilliance-40 and -64 scanners. Siemens uses a hybrid configuration that provides 32×0.6-mm and 20×1.2-mm sections on their Sensation-64 scanner. In addition, they use a flying focal spot along the z-axis that results in a second set of projectional data that is precisely offset by half the detector width. While this does not provide more than 32 detector rows, it does improve z-axis resolution and reduces artifacts. Toshiba uses a matrix configuration on their Aquilion-32 and -64, which provides 32 to 64×0.5 mm and 32 to 64×1 mm collimation, respectively. This new generation of 32- to 64-slice scanners will provide not only isotropic resolution and fast scan durations (<10 s for almost any body region), but will also improve cardiac gating options, which should further enhance the cardiac capabilities of these scanners.

Cone Beam Geometry and Data Reconstruction

Cone beam geometry is a problem that becomes important as the number of active detector channels grows (e.g., 16×1 mm) or the total active detector width increases (e.g., 4×5 mm). Under such conditions, the cone angle of the X-ray beam can no longer be assumed to pass in a parallel fashion from the tube to the detector [11]. As the tube rotates around the patient, structures may be "seen" by different detector rows during one rotation. If this incongruence is not corrected it can lead to considerable cone beam artifacts. Artifacts increase with higher pitch factors in most systems, but are less pronounced if a smaller field of view is used. Cone beam artifacts are most prominent at high-contrast interfaces that are almost parallel to the scan plane. They can best be seen on MPR. Typical regions that suffer most from such artifacts are the skull base or the ribs.

While linear interpolation algorithms are used to good advantage for four-slice systems, more advanced cone beam algorithms are necessary to cope with this problem and to reduce artifacts to a minimum.

Multislice Interpolation

For multislice interpolation at low cone angles, algorithms that are analogous to 180°LI and 360°LI from spiral CT can be used. They are called 180°MLI (multislice linear interpolation) and 360°MLI. For each projection angle, they use the projection data from the two detectors that are closest to the scanning plane (360°MLI only real trajectories, 180°MLI also virtual trajectories from the detector to the X-ray tube). Section profiles with these algorithms vary between those from conventional 180°LI and 360°LI spiral CT interpolation, but the dependence on the pitch factor is more complex because of the varying overlap of beam trajectories with increasing pitch.

Z-filter interpolation is the technique used to create a planar transaxial image from the projectional raw data in *four to eight-slice scanners*. Z-filter interpolation neglects the cone beam effect and therefore leads to an increased amount of artifact, as more than four detector rows are used. Z-filtering uses a similar concept as higher-order interpolation algorithms for conventional spiral CT [12, 13]. In addition to using two projections that are closest to the scan plane for image formation, adjacent projections (multipoint interpolation) are weighted according to their distance from the scan plane. Z-filtering is now available from all manufacturers and is used to control the width of the slice profile (section width, SW) of the reconstructed images. In principle, the only restraint is that the section width must be larger than the collimation.

Depending on the manufacturers, the slice profile and image noise may depend on the *pitch factor* (GE, Toshiba), while others (Siemens, Philips) maintain the section width independent of the pitch. While GE only allows for certain pitch factors (two choices for 4-slice scanners, four choices for 8- and 16-slice scanners), other manufacturers suggest preferential pitch factors (Philips, Toshiba) or arbitrary pitch factors (Siemens).

Cone Beam Interpolation

Real cone beam corrections are mandatory with 16 or more detector rows because cone beam artifacts increase substantially with wider detector arrays. Most of these algorithms are still being refined, and use various types of compensation techniques for the cone beam geometry. Variants of three-dimensional back projection (e.g., n-Pi reconstruction or COBRA, Philips; ConeView, Toshiba) should yield the fewest artifacts [11, 16]. Other techniques (e.g., Adaptive Multiple Plane Reconstruction, Siemens) shift the plane of interpolation from an axial orientation to an oblique position with a maximum angulation determined by the

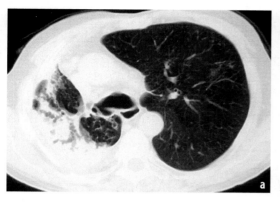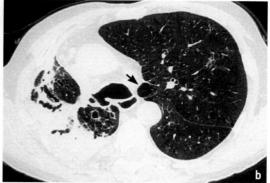

Fig. 5. Multislice scanning with thin sections (4×1-mm collimation) allows for reconstruction of conventional 5-mm-thick sections (**a**) as well as the reconstruction of thin (HRCT) sections (**b**) that can also be used to create a secondary raw data set for two- and three-dimensional imaging (compare with Fig. 6)

cone angle [17, 18]. This yields a set of oblique planes (as an intermediate step) that rotate with different z-positions. Interpolation between these oblique planes then creates axial, coronal, or arbitrarily oriented sections of any desired section width without necessarily having to produce a real reconstruction of an orthogonal three-dimensional data set.

Practical Approach

Scan Parameters

In MDCT the same acquired raw data set can be used to reconstruct two or more image data sets of varying thickness (Fig. 5). For this reason, one must distinguish between acquisition parameters (SC and TF) and reconstruction parameters (SW and RI).

To simplify notation, the *acquisition parameters* can be expressed as (N×SC/TF), where N is the number of detector rows. The table feed (TF) can be varied independently of the slice collimation (SC) as long as the pitch P is ≤2. However, the *definition of pitch* (P) varies between scanner manufacturers. Philips uses the definition preferred by most physicists and adopted as an international (IEC) standard, P=TF/(N×SC), where the table feed is related to the whole width of the active detector elements. GE, Siemens, and Toshiba, on the other hand, use P*=TF/SC (volume pitch, helical pitch, or beam pitch), at least on their four-slice units. This pitch definition relates the table feed to a single section width. The asterisk is used to differentiate the volume pitch from the international standard definition. The pitch P is now becoming increasingly more common as scanners with six or more detector rows enter the market.

The *reconstruction parameters* in MDCT can be expressed as one pair of numbers (SW/RI) per re-

constructed image data set. The slice width (SW) can be varied independently of how the data set has been acquired (at least in theory), as long as it is greater than the slice collimation (SC). If thick slices (SC) are used for scanning, it is not possible to reconstruct thinner slices (SW) for smaller detail later, while it is easy to reconstruct thick slices for clinical viewing if thin slices have been used for scanning. The reconstruction increment should then be about half the slice width in clinical practice, but need not be smaller than the pixel size (0.5–0.8-mm). More than one set of reconstructions (e.g., thin and thick sections) can be obtained from the same raw data set.

Choosing Scan Parameters

There are two different ways of choosing the scan parameters for MDCT (see Table 2). One is to preserve the workflow of single-slice spiral CT ("fast spiral acquisition"), while the other is to acquire a new isotropic three-dimensional volume that can be further processed ("volumetric imaging") [19].

For a *fast spiral acquisition*, axial sections of a thickness of about 5 mm are reconstructed for many indications in an analogous manner to conventional spiral CT. MPR and three-dimensional imaging are only carried out if necessary, depending on the clinical findings. This method is time- and cost-efficient, simple, and involves a known workflow [20]. However, the real opportunities inherent to MDCT are not optimally used. As 16-slice scanners become more widely available, this is unlikely to be the future method of choice.

Volumetric imaging relies on data acquisition using thin slices (small SC), which are then reconstructed to yield a nearly isotropic "*secondary raw data set*" that consists of thin, overlapping axial images [21]. Any other images (axial or multiplanar) that are required for clinical reporting can

Table 2. Suggested acquisition parameters for MDCT of the body (adapted from [19]). Note that the borders between fast spiral acquisitions and volumetric imaging blur for 16-slice units. For skeletal imaging, pitch factors lower than 1 should be used to minimize artifacts on multiplanar reformation

Scanner type	Fast spiral scanning			Volumetric imaging		
	SC (mm)	TF (mm)	P	SC (mm)	TF (mm)	P
4-slice (GE)	2.5	15	1.5	1.25	7.5	1.5
4-slice (Philips)	2.5	15	1.5	1	6	1.5
4-slice (Siemens)	2.5	15	1.5	1	6	1.5
4-slice (Toshiba)	2–3	11–16.5	1.375	1	5.5	1.375
6-slice (Siemens)	3	22.5	1.5	1	9	1.5
8-slice (GE)	2.5	27	1.35	1.25	13.5	1.35
10-slice (Siemens)	1.5	22.5	1.5	0.75	11.25	1.5
16-slice (GE)	1.25	27.5	1.375	0.625	13.75	1.375
16-slice (Philips)	1.5	30	1.25	0.75	15	1.25
16-slice (Siemens)	1.5	36	1.5	0.75	18	1.5
16-slice (Toshiba)	2	30	0.9375	0.5–1	11.5–23	1.4375
Indication						
Neck	Standard, lymph node staging			Tumor staging		
Chest	Metastases, mediastinum			Tumor staging, interstitial disease		
Abdomen	Standard abdomen, liver (non-contrast), kidneys (benign disease)			Pancreas, liver, biliary system, bowel, preoperative evaluation		
CTA	Aorta, dyspneic patients, veins			Carotids, pulmonary vessels, abdominal arteries		
Skeleton	Pelvis, lumbar spine, long bones			Small joints, small bones, C- and T-spine		

SC=slice collimation, *TF*=table feed/rotation, *P*=pitch=TF/($n×$SC), *n*=number of active detector rows

subsequently be constructed from this secondary raw data set.

Most frequently 3- to 6-mm axial sections are reconstructed for clinical viewing, which is very similar to the sections reconstructed from a fast spiral acquisition. However, the "added value" of multislice scanning is provided by coronal or sagittal multiplanar reformations, curved planar reformations, or reformations of arbitrary orientation through the data volume. Which of these sections are best suited, will depend on the clinical indication. Further processing such as various three-dimensional rendering techniques (volume rendering or maximum intensity projections) may prove beneficial, especially when it comes to the display of vascular or skeletal structures. Increasing the thickness of the MPR improves the signal-to-noise ratio (SNR). The thickness needed for MPR depends on the indication.

Volumetric imaging relies on a completely new workflow that is more similar to MRI than conventional CT techniques. Only when the scanner and workstation software can handle large amounts of data quickly and easily will volumetric imaging become a time- and cost-effective alternative to fast spiral scanning. However, volumetric imaging makes optimum use of MDCT capabilities (Fig. 6) and is already well suited to complex cases, particularly vascular or skeletal studies. Scanner manufacturers realize that volumetric imaging is likely to become the preferred method in the future and are working to improve the workflow for this situation.

Future Trends

There are a number of main avenues for technical improvement in multislice scanning.

1. *Faster rotation speed* of the X-ray tube will allow for better cardiac imaging. In this context, combinations of electron beam CT with multislice detectors may be seen in the future.

2. *Wider detectors* with more detector rows will allow for more coverage per rotation. However, if the irradiated volume becomes too large, scattered radiation can substantially reduce image quality. Scatter correction, however, requires an additional dose for adequate SNR. For this reason, some manufacturers consider very wide detectors mainly for use in a hybrid mode, in which the CT scanner can be used also for fluoroscopy while the tube stands still.

3. *Higher isotropic resolution* will be possible with smaller detector elements. Preliminary studies using area detectors or "micro-CT" units have been

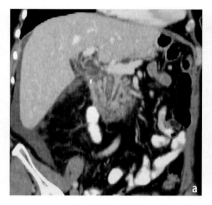
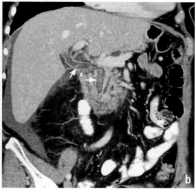

Fig. 6. Coronal images of the common bile duct reformatted from 3-mm-thick axial sections (**a**) and 1.25-mm-thick sections (**b**). Note the increase in clarity of the images derived from the thinner slices, where hyperdense material (*arrows*) can be seen in the common bile duct of this patient with hemobilia

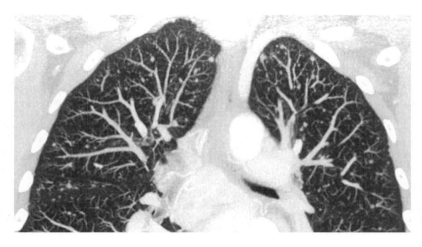

Fig. 7. Coronal thin-slab maximum intensity projection (MIP) in a patient with multiple tiny pulmonary metastases from medullary thyroid cancer. Data were acquired with 40×0.625-mm collimation and a matrix size of 768^2, resulting in isotropic 0.45-mm resolution

very successful for small animal experiments and explanted organs. Because image noise increases extremely rapidly (with a power of 2), dose requirements for constant SNR increase even faster (with a power of 4). This means that one needs $2^4(=16)$ times more dose to increase resolution from 1 mm^3 to 0.5 mm^3. This will substantially restrict possible applications in body CT imaging in humans. Most manufacturers have now chosen detector widths between 0.5 and 0.625 mm, resulting in minimum effective section widths of 0.6–0.67 mm. The resulting spatial resolution in high-contrast phantoms is in the range of 0.4 mm in the z-direction and 0.4–0.6 mm in the scan plane (Fig. 7).

4. *Larger image matrices* are required in order to take advantage of this improved spatial resolution. For a standard chest or abdomen, a FOV of 300–400 mm is chosen, resulting in pixel sizes of 0.6–0.8 mm. In order to take advantage of the improved resolution, larger matrices (e.g., 768^2 or $1,024^2$) are required (Fig. 7).

5. *Functional imaging* and *perfusion imaging* will be of interest if low-dose techniques can be combined with wider detectors. Already brain perfusion in stroke patients is a major clinical indication. Philips, for example, will provide a "jog mode" on their 40-slice unit, in which the scanner alternates between two table positions and thus is able to cover a range of 80 mm.

6. *Image processing* and *computer-aided diagnosis* tools are being developed that will help with tedious imaging tasks such as nodule detection, polyp detection, and volume quantification. They are a prerequisite for bronchial cancer or colon cancer screening if performed on a population basis. In addition, volumetric analysis will present new opportunities for treatment and follow-up of patients with malignant disease, thus allowing for fine-tuning and individualized therapy.

References

1. Klingenbeck-Regn K, Schaller S, Flohr T et al (1999) Subsecond multi-slice computed tomography: basics and applications. Eur J Radiol 31:110-124
2. Hu H, He HD, Foley WD et al (2000) Four multidetector-row helical CT: image quality and volume coverage speed. Radiology 215:55-62
3. Rubin GD, Shiau MC, Leung AN et al (2000) Aorta and iliac arteries: single versus multiple detector-row helical CT angiography. Radiology 215:670-676
4. Mahesh M (2002) The AAPM/RSNA physics tutorial for residents: search for isotropic resolution in CT from conventional through multiple-row detector. Radiographics 22:949-962
5. Flohr T, Stierstorfer K, Bruder H et al (2002) New technical developments in multislice CT. 1. Approaching isotropic resolution with sub-millimeter 16-slice scanning. Rofo Fortschr Geb Rontgenstr Neuen Bildgeb Verfahr 174:839-845
6. Rubin GD (2000) Data explosion: the challenge of multidetector row CT. Eur J Radiol 36:74-80
7. Prokop M (2003) Radiation exposure and image quality. In: Prokop M, Galanski M (eds) Spiral and multislice computed tomography of the body. Thieme, Stuttgart, pp 131-160
8. McCollough CH, Zink FE (1999) Performance evaluation of a multi-slice CT system. Med Phys 26:2223-2230
9. Prokop M (2003) General principles of MDCT. Eur J Radiol 45 [Suppl 1]:S4-S10
10. Weidekamm C, Prokop M, Herold C (2002) Low kVp settings improve contrast enhancement and reduce radiation exposure in spiral CT of pulmonary emboli. Eur Radiol 12 [Suppl]:149
11. Proksa R, Kohler T, Grass M et al (2000) The n-PI-method for helical cone-beam CT. IEEE Trans Med Imaging 19:848-863
12. Fuchs T, Krause J, Schaller S et al (2000) Spiral interpolation algorithms for multislice spiral CT. II. Measurement and evaluation of slice sensitivity profiles and noise at a clinical multislice system. IEEE Trans Med Imaging 19:835-847
13. Taguchi K, Aradate H (1998) Algorithm for image reconstruction in multi-slice helical CT. Med Phys 25:550-553
14. Hsieh J (2001) Investigation of the slice-sensitivity profile for step-and-shoot mode multi-slice computed tomogaphy. Med Phys 28:491-497
15. Wang G, Vannier MW (1999) The effect of pitch in multislice spiral/helical CT. Med Phys 26:2648-2653
16. Taguchi K, Zeng GL, Gullberg GT (2001) Cone-beam image reconstruction using spherical harmonics. Phys Med Biol 46:N127-N138
17. Kachelriess M, Schaller S, Kalender WA (2000) Advanced single-slice rebinning in cone-beam spiral CT. Med Phys 27:574-572
18. Schaller S, Stierstorfer K, Bruder H, et al (2001) Novel approximate approach for high quality image reconstruction in helical cone-beam CT at arbitrary pitch. Proc SPIE 4322:113-127
19. Prokop M (2003) Optimization of scanning technique. In: Prokop M, Galanski M (eds) Spiral and multislice computed tomography of the body. Thieme, Stuttgart, pp 109-130
20. Jhaveri KS, Saini S, Levine LA et al (2001) Effect of multislice CT technology on scanner productivity. AJR 177:769-772
21. Prokop M (2003) Image processing and display techniques. In: Prokop M, Galanski M (eds) Spiral and multislice computed tomography of the body. Thieme, Stuttgart, pp 45-82

I.2

Contrast Medium Administration and Scan Timing for MDCT

Jay P. Heiken and Kyongtae T. Bae

Introduction

As computed tomography (CT) technology has evolved from single-slice imaging to 4- and 16-slice scanners, the speed at which the patient is passed through the gantry has increased up to eight-fold, depending on the technique used (Table 1). Therefore, the time to scan a body part or the entire body has been reduced substantially. For example, a chest scan that used to require 36 s on a single-slice scanner with 3-mm collimation now takes 5–10 s on a 16-slice scanner with 0.625 - 1.5 mm detector collimation; a chest–abdomen–pelvis examination, which was not really feasible with single-slice scanners (requiring 80 s), is now possible in 10-20 s.

The markedly reduced scan durations for multidetector–row CT (MDCT) examinations have made scan timing more critical than for single-detector CT. At the same time, these short scan times have provided radiologists with an opportunity to improve contrast enhancement with MDCT. It is therefore important for radiologists and technologists to: (1) understand the factors that determine both the timing and magnitude of arterial and hepatic parenchymal contrast enhancement for CT, and (2) identify the modifications needed to optimize contrast enhancement for 4-, 8-, 16-, and the new 64-row MDCT scanners.

Table 1. Changes in table feed with evolution in CT technology

Detector configuration	Table feed, mm/s
Single row (3-5 mm detector collimation)	8
4 detector rows (1-mm detector collimation)	10
4 detector rows (2.5-mm detector collimation)	24
16 detector rows (0.75-mm detector collimation)	30
16 detector rows (1.5-mm detector collimation)	60

Scan Timing

Technical Factors

The most important technical factor that affects scan timing is the duration of contrast medium injection [1-3], which is determined by the volume of contrast medium and the rate at which it is administered. In patients with normal cardiac output, peak arterial contrast enhancement is achieved shortly after the termination of injection of contrast medium [4]. As the contrast medium volume increases, the time it takes to reach the peaks of arterial and hepatic parenchymal contrast enhancement also increases (Fig. 1) [5]. Conversely, an increase in injection rate results in a shorter time to peak enhancement (Fig. 2) [5]. Therefore, a short injection duration (i.e., small volume or high injection rate) results in earlier peak arterial and hepatic parenchymal enhancement, which requires a short scan delay. A long injection duration (i.e., large volume or low injection rate) results in later peak enhancement, requiring a long scan delay.

Patient-Related Factors

The most important patient-related factor that affects scan timing is cardiac output [6]. Decreased cardiac output (i.e., increased cardiovascular transit time) results in delayed arrival of the contrast bolus in the aorta, which leads to delayed arterial and hepatic parenchymal enhancement (Fig. 3). Because of substantial variation in cardiac output among patients, it is important to individualize the scan delay for imaging studies in which scan timing is critical, e.g., CT angiography (CTA). Scan delay can be individualized by using a test bolus [7, 8] or a bolus-tracking software program [9].

The test bolus method (Fig. 4) is the more commonly used technique, but it must be adapted for use with the faster scanners. Typically, we give a

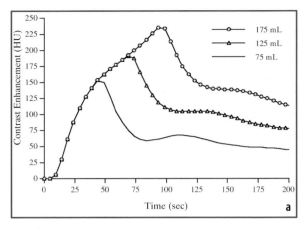
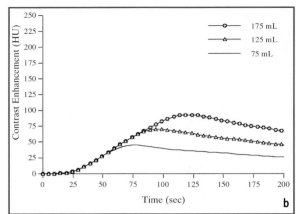

Fig. 1a, b. Simulated contrast enhancement curves with three different contrast medium volumes. Simulated enhancement curves of **a** the aorta and **b** the liver based on a hypothetical adult male with a fixed height (5'8" or 173 cm) and body weight (150 lb or 68 kg), subject to injection of 75, 125, and 175 ml of 320 mg I/ml contrast medium at 2 ml/s. The time to peak enhancement and the magnitude of peak enhancement increase with increased contrast medium volume. (Reprinted from [28])

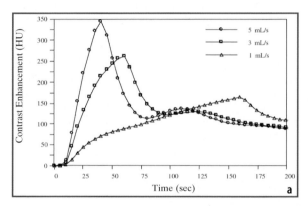
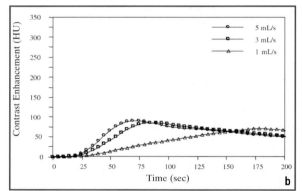

Fig. 2a, b. Simulated contrast enhancement curves with three different contrast medium injection rates. Simulated enhancement curves of **a** the aorta and **b** the liver based on a hypothetical adult male with a fixed height (5'8" or 173 cm) and body weight (150 lb or 68 kg), subject to 150 ml of 320 mg I/ml contrast medium injected at 1, 3, and 5 ml/s. The curves show that for a constant volume of contrast medium, as the rate of injection increases, the time it takes to reach the peak of enhancement decreases and the magnitude of peak enhancement increases. (Reprinted from [29])

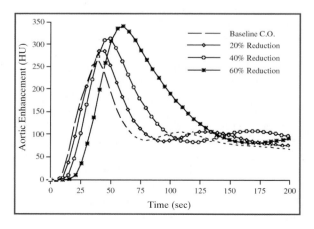

Fig. 3. Simulated contrast enhancement curves at baseline and reduced cardiac outputs. Simulated enhancement curves of the aorta based on a hypothetical adult male with a fixed height (5'8" or 173 cm) and body weight (150 lb or 68 kg), subject to injection of 120 ml of 320 mg I/ml contrast medium at 4 ml/s. A set of aortic and hepatic contrast enhancement curves were generated from the model by reducing the baseline cardiac output, i.e. 6500 ml/min, by 20%, 40%, and 60%. (Reprinted from [29])

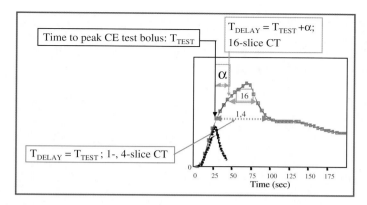

Fig. 4. Test bolus method for individualizing the scan delay. On single- or 4-detector-row scanners, the scan delay (the time between the start of contrast medium administration and that of scanning) is determined as the time necessary for aortic enhancement to peak after a small bolus injection of contrast medium. With faster scanners, scanning must be delayed further (α) if imaging is to be performed during the peak enhancement of the aorta. *Horizontal lines*, scanning period for 1- or 4-detector-row scanners (*red*) and for 16-detector-row scanners (*blue*)

small bolus (15–20 ml) of contrast medium at the rate to be used for the diagnostic examination, and we determine when aortic enhancement peaks. For single- and 4-detector-row scanners, the time of peak aortic enhancement after a small bolus is used as the scan delay for the diagnostic examination; this assures that diagnostic scanning is performed during the peak of aortic enhancement after administration of a full bolus of contrast medium. However, with faster scanners and thus shorter scan durations, scanning must be delayed even further if imaging is to be performed during the peak of aortic enhancement. This is done by adding an additional delay (α) to that calculated on the basis of the test bolus. The test bolus method is effective for determining the scan delay for a single patient, but it is not an efficient method because it requires an additional volume of contrast medium and is time-consuming.

A more efficient and elegant method to determine the correct timing of scanning after contrast medium administration involves the use of bolus-tracking software with a region of interest (ROI) placed over the aorta (Fig. 5). A regular bolus of

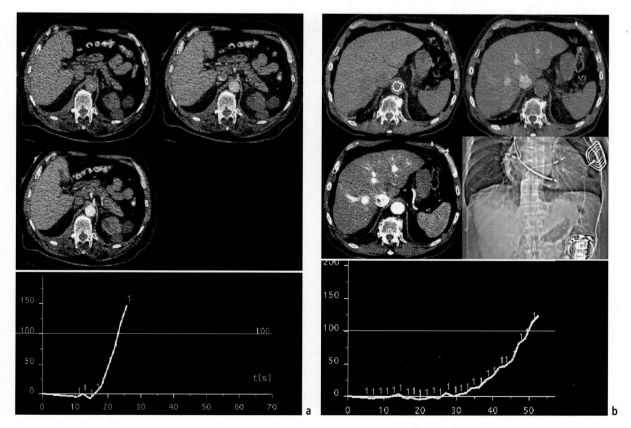

Fig. 5a, b. Determination of scan delay using bolus-tracking software. **a** Patient with normal cardiac output: the 100 HU threshold is reached at about 25 s. **b** Patient with poor cardiac output: the 100 HU threshold is not reached until 50 s after bolus injection. Had this examination been started at 25 s (the scan delay typically used for patients with normal cardiac output), the bolus would have been missed and imaging would have been performed too early

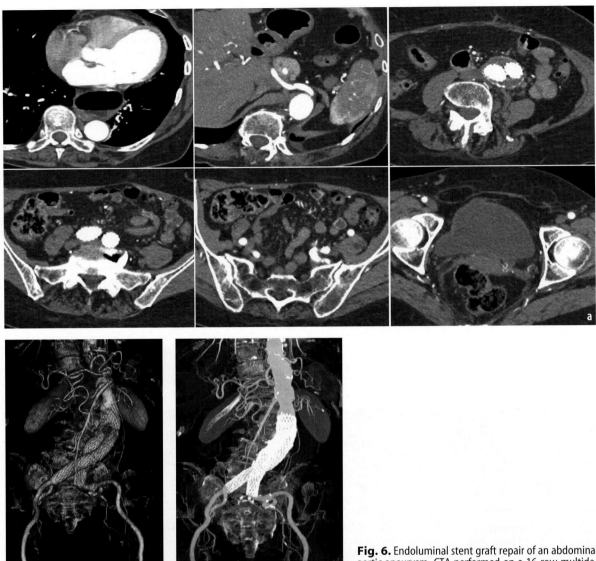

Fig. 6. Endoluminal stent graft repair of an abdominal aortic aneurysm. CTA performed on a 16-row multidetector CT scanner using only 75 ml of contrast medium. **a** Transaxial image. **b** Volume-rendered image. **c** Maximum intensity projection image

contrast medium is administered and, approximately 10 s after the bolus injection is begun, low-dose monitoring scans are made to track enhancement in the aorta. When a predetermined threshold (e.g. 100 HU) is reached, regular scanning is triggered. This method makes it possible to appropriately determine the scan delay for individual patients with only a single injection of contrast medium.

Increasing the scan delay is one approach to optimizing scan timing when working with faster CT scanners. Alternatively, with 8- and 16-row MDCT, one can take advantage of the very short scan durations by reducing the volume of contrast medium administered; for example, using a 16-detector-row scanner, excellent images can be obtained using only 75 ml of iodinated contrast medium

(Fig. 6). The new 64-row scanner may allow a further reduction in the volume of contrast medium. Nonetheless, the use of smaller volumes of contrast medium may require that the scanning protocol be optimized to overcome the possibility of reduced enhancement.

Contrast Enhancement Magnitude

Technical Factors

Arterial Enhancement. The magnitude of arterial enhancement is determined by the rate of iodine delivery into the vascular system. The rate of iodine delivery depends upon three factors: (1) the

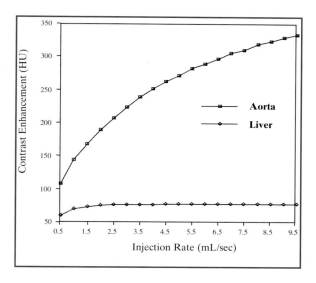

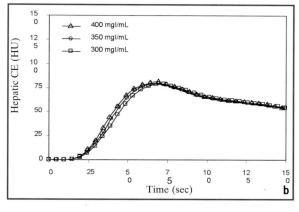

Fig. 7. Effect of contrast medium injection rate on the magnitude of peak contrast enhancement (from simulated contrast enhancement curves). Peak aortic and hepatic contrast enhancements at different injection rates are simulated based on a hypothetical adult male with a fixed height (5'8" or 173 cm) and body weight (150 lb or 68 kg), subject to injection of 120 ml of 320 mgI/ml contrast medium. (Reprinted from [1])

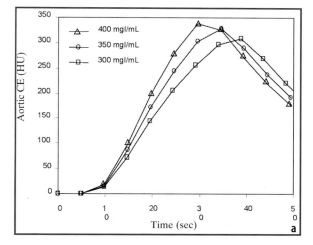

Fig. 8a, b. Simulated contrast enhancement curves with a fixed amount of iodine mass but three different contrast medium concentrations injected at a constant rate. Simulated enhancement curves of **a** the aorta and **b** liver based on a hypothetical adult male with a fixed height (5'8" or 173 cm) and body weight (150 lb or 68 kg), subject to 5 ml/s injection of the same amount of iodine mass but at three different concentrations and volumes: 300 mg I/ml, 140 ml; 350 mg I/ml, 120 ml; and 400 mg I/ml, 105 ml. The aortic and hepatic time-enhancement curves demonstrate that the use of high-concentration contrast material is associated with earlier and greater peak aortic enhancement. The effect on hepatic parenchymal enhancement is minimal. (Reprinted from [29])

concentration of iodine in the contrast medium, (2) the injection rate (Fig. 7), and (3) the injection volume (primarily through recirculation of contrast medium already in the vascular system). Increases in iodine concentration [10], injection rate [1, 11], and volume [10] all result in increased arterial enhancement. Use of contrast material with a higher iodine concentration produces more aortic contrast enhancement, even if the total iodine dose and injection rate are unchanged, by virtue of increasing the rate of iodine delivery to the vascular system (Fig. 8). When the contrast medium volume is reduced for CTA with 8- and 16-row (and in future 64-row) MDCT, an increased injection rate and high iodine concentration can compensate for the somewhat decreased magnitude of aortic en-

hancement achieved with the smaller contrast medium volume.

Hepatic Parenchymal Enhancement. Hepatic parenchymal enhancement is determined by the total iodine dose administered [3, 12–18], which in turn is determined by the contrast medium volume and iodine concentration. Use of contrast material with a higher iodine concentration improves hepatic parenchymal enhancement to the extent that it increases overall iodine dose [19]. The injection rate plays a more limited role in hepatic parenchymal contrast enhancement (Fig. 7); the concentration of iodine in the contrast medium has little effect on hepatic parenchymal enhancement if the total dose is constant (Fig. 8).

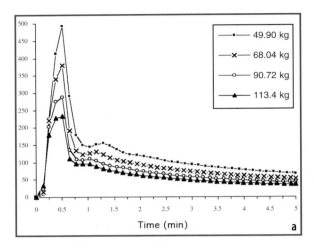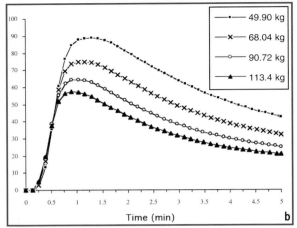

Fig. 9a, b. Simulated contrast enhancement curves with four different body weights. Simulated enhancement curves of **a** the aorta and **b** liver based on a hypothetical adult male with a fixed height (5'8″ or 173 cm) and varying body weight (110, 160, 200, and 260 lb), subject to injection of 125 ml of 320 mg I/ml contrast medium at 5 ml/s. The magnitude of contrast enhancement is inversely proportional to the body weight. (Reprinted from [28])

Although a rapid injection rate (e.g. 5 ml/s) does not increase the magnitude of hepatic parenchymal enhancement compared with an intermediate injection rate (e.g. 2–3 ml/s), it does increase the magnitude of hepatic arterial enhancement and it separates the peaks of hepatic arterial and hepatic parenchymal enhancement [1], thus improving detection of hypervascular liver masses [20]. Similarly, a rapid injection rate increases pancreatic parenchymal enhancement [21, 22]. Therefore a rapid injection rate is useful for dedicated hepatic and pancreatic imaging protocols. Use of higher-concentration contrast material increases tumor-to-liver contrast of hepatocellular carcinoma during the arterial phase of enhancement, and therefore is also useful for detecting hypervascular liver masses [23].

Patient-Related Factors

The most important patient-related factor that affects the magnitude of both arterial and hepatic parenchymal contrast enhancement is body weight [14, 24], which is inversely related to the magnitude of enhancement. In larger, heavier patients, less contrast enhancement is achieved for a given iodine dose compared with smaller patients (Fig. 9). Therefore, when imaging heavy patients, one should consider modifying the contrast administration protocol by increasing the contrast medium concentration, volume, or injection rate.

Scanning Protocol Modifications for MDCT

As stated previously, with MDCT, the shorter scan duration requires a longer scan delay to image during the peak parenchymal enhancement (Fig. 10). For CT angiography a preferable alternative to delayed imaging with the standard injection protocol is to reduce the volume of contrast medium. With a smaller volume, we can image during the peak of

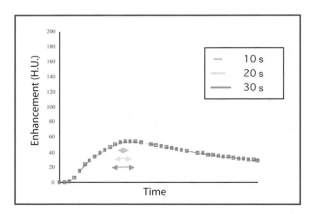

Fig. 10. Timing of hepatic CT scanning as a function of parenchymal enhancement kinetics and speed of the CT scanner. With faster scanners, scanning is started later after the administration of contrast medium and is performed for a shorter period

aortic enhancement using a scan delay similar to that of the traditional injection protocol. While a reduced volume of contrast medium is advantageous for many reasons, the magnitude of peak contrast enhancement is reduced. This disadvantage may be compensated for by injecting at a faster rate or by using a contrast medium with an increased iodine concentration.

Saline Flush

Use of a saline flush immediately after contrast medium injection has several advantages. It increases peak aortic enhancement by: (1) pushing into the cardiovascular system contrast material that otherwise would be left in the injection tubing, and (2) improving bolus geometry by limiting contrast medium dispersion. Thus, when a saline flush is employed, one can achieve an equivalent magnitude of contrast enhancement with a smaller contrast medium volume [25-27]. An additional advantage of a saline flush is that it minimizes streak artifact from dense contrast material in the brachiocephalic vein and superior vena cava on thoracic CT examinations [25, 26].

Conclusions

With MDCT, scan timing is even more critical than with single-detector CT, and will continue to be so as the number of detector rows increases to 32 and 64. For CTA, in which scan timing is particularly critical, the scan delay can be accurately determined by use of a test bolus or bolus-tracking software.

The magnitude of arterial enhancement is determined primarily by iodine flux (g/s) and therefore is strongly and directly correlated with injection rate and contrast medium concentration. With fast scanners (e.g., 8 and 16 detector rows), the short scan duration requires a longer scan delay for CTA and hepatic parenchymal imaging. Alternatively, we can modify the injection protocol, taking into consideration the type of imaging to be performed. For arterial imaging, it is possible to decrease the volume of contrast medium when using rapid injection rates and high contrast medium concentrations. However, for hepatic parenchymal imaging, the magnitude of enhancement is mainly determined by the total iodine dose, and injection rate makes only a limited contribution. Therefore, when performing hepatic imaging with fast CT scanners, only limited reduction of iodine dose is feasible. Contrast volume can be reduced to a greater extent if a higher concentration contrast medium is used.

References

1. Bae KT, Heiken JP, Brink JA (1998) Aortic and hepatic peak enhancement at CT: effect of contrast medium injection rate, pharmacokinetic analysis and experimental porcine model. Radiology 206:455-464
2. Heiken JP, Brink JA, McClennan BL et al (1993) Dynamic contrast-enhanced CT of the liver: comparison of contrast medium injection rates and uniphasic and biphasic injection protocols. Radiology 187:327-331
3. Chambers TP, Baron RL, Lush RM (1994) Hepatic CT enhancement. Part I. Alterations in the volume of contrast material within the same patients. Radiology 193:513-517
4. Bae KT (2003) Peak contrast enhancement in CT and MR angiography: when does it occur and why? Pharmacokinetic study in a porcine model. Radiology 227:809-816
5. Han JK, Kim AY, Lee KY et al (2000) Factors influencing vascular and hepatic enhancement at CT: experimental study on injection protocol using a canine model. J Comput Assist Tomogr 24:400-406
6. Bae KT, Heiken JP, Brink JA (1998) Aortic and hepatic contrast medium enhancement at CT. II. Effect of reduced cardiac output in a porcine model. Radiology 207:657-662
7. Van Hoe L, Marchal G, Baert AL et al (1995) Determination of scan delay-time in spiral CT-angiography: utility of a test bolus injection. J Comput Assist Tomogr 19:216-220
8. Hittmair K, Fleischmann D (2001) Accuracy of predicting and controlling time-dependent aortic enhancement from a test bolus injection. J Comput Assist Tomogr 25:287-294
9. Silverman PM, Roberts, S, Tefft MC et al (1995) Helical CT of the liver: clinical application of an automated computer technique, SmartPrep, for obtaining images with optimal contrast enhancement. AJR Am J Roentgenol 165:73-78
10. Fleischmann D (2002) Present and future trends in multiple detector-row CT applications: CT angiography. Eur Radiol 12[Suppl 2]:S11-16
11. Fleischmann D (2003) Use of high-concentration contrast media in multi-detector row CT: principles and rationale. Eur Radiol 13[Suppl 5]:M14-M20
12. Berland LL, Lee JY (1988) Comparison of contrast media injection rates and volumes for hepatic dynamic incremented computed tomography. Invest Radiol 23:918-922
13. Dean PB, Violante MR, Mahoney JA (1980) Hepatic CT contrast enhancement: effect of dose, duration of infusion and time elapsed following infusion. Invest Radiol 15:158-161
14. Heiken JP, Brink JA, McClennan BL et al (1995) Dynamic incremental CT: effect of volume and concentration of contrast material and patient weight on hepatic enhancement. Radiology 195:353-357
15. Claussen CD, Banzer D, Pfretzschner C et al (1984) Bolus geometry and dynamics after intravenous contrast medium injection. Radiology 153:365-368
16. Chambers TP, Baron RL, Lush RM (1994) Hepatic CT enhancement. II. Alterations in contrast material volume and rate of injection within the same patients. Radiology 193:518-522

17. Harmon BH, Berland LL, Lee JY (1992) Effect of varying rates of low-osmolarity contrast media injection for hepatic CT: correlation with indocyanine green transit time. Radiology 184:379-382

18. Garcia P, Genin G, Bret PM et al (1999) Hepatic CT enhancement: effects of the rate and volume of contrast medium injection in an animal model. Abdom Imaging 24:597-603

19. Furuta A, Ito K, Fujita T et al (2004) Hepatic enhancement in multiphasic contrast-enhanced MD-CT: comparison of high- and low-iodine-concentration contrast medium in same patients with chronic liver disease. AJR Am J Roentgenol 183:157-162

20. Kim T, Murakami T, Takahashi S et al (1998) Effect of injection rates of contrast material on arterial phase hepatic CT. AJR Am J Roentgenol 171:429-432

21. Tublin ME, Tessler FN, Cheng SL et al (1999) Effect of injection rate of contrast medium on pancreatic and hepatic helical CT. Radiology 210:97-101

22. Kim T, Murakami T, Takahashi S et al (1999) Pancreatic CT imaging: effects of different injection rates and doses of contrast material. Radiology 212:219-225

23. Awai K, Takada K, Onishi H (2002) Aortic and hepatic enhancement and tumor-to-liver contrast: analysis of the effect of different concentrations of contrast material at multidetector-row helical CT. Radiology 224:757-763

24. Kormano M, Partanen K, Soimakallio S (1983) Dynamic contrast enhancement of the upper abdomen: effect of contrast medium and body weight. Invest Radiol 18:364-367

25. Hopper KD, Mosher TJ, Kasales CJ et al (1997) Thoracic spiral CT: delivery of contrast material pushed with injectable saline solution in a power injector. Radiology 205:269-271

26. Haage P, Schmitz-Rode T, Hübner D et al (2000) Reduction of contrast material dose and artifacts by a saline flush using a double power injector in helical CT of the thorax. AJR Am J Roentgenol 174:1049-1053

27. Dorio PJ, Lee FT, Henseler KP et al (2003) Using a saline chaser to decrease contrast media in abdominal CT. AJR Am J Roentgenol 180:929-934

28. Bae KT, Heiken JP (2000) Computer modeling approach to contrast medium administration and scan timing for multislice CT. In: Marincek B, Ros PR, Reiser M, Baker ME (eds) Multislice CT: a practical guide. Springer pp 28-36

29. Bae KT (2003) Technical aspects of contrast delivery in advanced CT. Appl Radiol 32[Suppl]:12-19

SECTION II

Abdominal Imaging

II

Introduction

Bernard E. Van Beers

Multidetector-row helical computed tomography (MDCT) has the potential to improve the diagnostic assessment of the abdomen. CT colonography is an emerging method to screen for colonic polyps [1] and CT remains one of the main diagnostic methods for imaging the hepatobiliary system and the pancreas. The high speed of MDCT can be used to cover larger anatomical volumes, to increase the spatial resolution along the z-axis, and to decrease the acquisition time. With a short acquisition time, the different phases of enhancement in the liver and pancreas can be easily separated, and with thin collimation, high-quality multiplanar and three-dimensional images can be obtained. This may be particularly important to assess vascular invasion in pancreatic tumors [2].

Optimization of the injection of contrast media in MDCT requires an understanding of contrast media dynamics. The magnitude of enhancement of an organ is determined by the net iodine flux into the organ. During the early phase after injection, enhancement depends on both intrinsic factors, i.e., circulation time and central volume, and extrinsic factors, i.e., contrast medium volume, contrast medium concentration, and injection rate. Increasing the injection rate improves the enhancement of the arteries and organs with arterial perfusion, such as the pancreas, by increasing the iodine flux into these organs. In contrast, increasing the injection rate has little effect on the enhancement of the liver, which is mainly perfused through the portal vein. Indeed, the dispersion of the bolus in an additional capillary bed before reaching the liver through the portal vein has a buffering effect opposing that of the increased injection rate. Therefore, a rapid injection rate (5 ml/s) does not increase the magnitude of hepatic enhancement compared with an intermediate rate (2–3 ml/s) [3]. As the liver enhancement depends only on the contrast agent volume and concentration, higher-concentration contrast agents should be used to improve the enhancement of the liver, without increasing the volume of the contrast agent [4, 5]. In contrast, the enhancement of vessels, pancreas, and hypervascular liver tumors can be improved by increasing the injection rate or the concentration of the contrast agent [6].

In addition, parenchymal and vascular enhancement can be improved by using a double-syringe injector with saline flush following contrast material bolus [7]. This improvement is explained by the fact that the saline pushes the contrast material that otherwise would be retained in the brachial vein and the superior vena cava.

With MDCT, automated coordination of contrast material arrival and initiation of scanning is useful. For arterial-phase imaging, CT examinations are triggered after aortic enhancement of 150 HU. Triggering can also be performed during the hepatic portal venous phase at 55-HU hepatic enhancement [8].

In conclusion, optimization of the scanning technique and contrast material injection is important for MDCT of the abdomen. The protocols will continue to evolve with the development of new CT scanners with increased detector rows.

References

1. Pickhardt PJ, Choi JR, Hwang I et al (2003) Computed tomographic virtual colonoscopy to screen for colorectal neoplasia in asymptomatic adults. N Engl J Med 349:2191-2200
2. Fenchel S, Boll DT, Fleiter TR et al (2003) Multislice helical CT of the pancreas and spleen. Eur J Radiol 4:S59-S7
3. Bae KT, Heiken JP, Brink JA (1998) Aortic and hepatic peak enhancement at CT: effect of contrast medium injection rate. Pharmacokinetic analysis and experimental porcine model. Radiology 206:455-464

4. Brink JA (2003) Use of high concentration contrast media (HCCM): principles and rationale. Body CT. Eur J Radiol 45:S53-S58
5. Furuta A, Ito K, Fujita T et al (2004) Hepatic enhancement in multiphasic contrast-enhanced MD-CT: comparison of high- and low-iodine-concentration contrast medium in same patients with chronic liver disease. AJR Am J Roentgenol 183:157-162
6. Awai K, Takada K, Onishi H et al (2002) Aortic and hepatic enhancement and tumor-to-liver contrast: analysis of the effect of different concentrations of contrast material at multi-detector row helical CT. Radiology 224:757-763
7. Schoellnast H, Tillich M, Deutschmann HA et al (2004) Improvement of parenchymal and vascular enhancement using saline flush and power injection for multiple-detector-row abdominal CT. Eur Radiol 14:659-664
8. Saini S (2004) Multi-detector row CT: principles and practice for abdominal applications. Radiology 223:323-327

II.1

Imaging Benign and Metastatic Liver Tumors with MDCT

Pierre-Jean Valette, Frank Pilleul and Arielle Crombé-Ternamian

Introduction

Multidetector-row computed tomography (MDCT) is a state of the art technology that provides high-resolution diagnostic images and facilitates the generation of three-dimensional displays. Whether these enhanced imaging capabilities will translate into improved diagnosis of liver neoplasms is currently an area of investigation, requiring both technical optimization of the technique and attention to the clinical objectives of the imaging examination.

The improved resolution of MDCT is achieved not only by the use of multiple detectors but also by the imaging protocol that involves thinner slices and faster acquisition times. These technical characteristics render the MDCT modality particularly sensitive to the way contrast medium is administered, so that clinicians face new challenges in optimizing the contrast medium injection and the image acquisition protocols for specific clinical situations.

The clinical objectives of a diagnostic imaging examination of the liver depend on the type of lesion expected. In patients with suspected benign liver tumors, imaging serves to characterize the lesion in order to confidently formulate a diagnostic hypothesis; in such cases an imaging modality with high specificity is essential. In contrast, in patients with a known primary malignancy of non-hepatic tissue, imaging is used to determine the presence or absence of secondary hepatic metastases; in these cases, the imaging modality must offer high sensitivity as well as high negative predictive value.

Technical Aspects of MDCT

The ability to detect liver lesions after the administration of contrast medium depends on the extent to which lesions differ from normal liver tissue in taking up the contrast agent. Hypervascular tumors take up more contrast agent than normal tissue and thus appear brighter (hyperintense), whereas hypovascular lesions are darker (hypointense). Diagnostic information is also obtained from the pattern of enhancement of hypervascular tumors compared to that of the surrounding liver tissue.

As a result of the liver's dual blood supply, contrast-enhanced imaging of the liver is performed during several vascular phases defined in relation to the moment when contrast medium is injected (Fig. 1) [1, 2]. Within the first 20 s after an intravenous bolus injection, there is relatively little effect of contrast agent on the imaging appearance of liver tissue; this *early arterial phase* is useful in defining the hepatic arterial anatomy before surgery but has little value in detecting and characterizing tumors. Between 30 and 35 s, during the *late arterial phase*, a sufficient amount of the contrast medium bolus reaches the liver and results in an enhanced appearance of liver tissues; areas of increased vascular density such as hypervascular lesions appear more conspicuous and hyperintense to the surrounding liver tissue. After 1 min, contrast agent is also brought to the liver by the portal venous blood supply; during this *portal venous phase* the distinction between normal liver tissue and hypervascular lesions is lost, while hypovascular lesions become clearly visible as areas that are hypointense to normal tissue. Imaging during the *late phase*, after several minutes, is useful to demonstrate persistent enhancement of some tumors (e.g., hemangiomas) and fibrotic lesions when contrast agent has been eliminated from normal liver tissue. Since the increased vascularity of tumors, relative to normal tissue, develops from the arterial blood supply, these lesions are best imaged during the brief arterial phase after the administration of contrast medium; therefore, it is important to carefully time the image acquisition

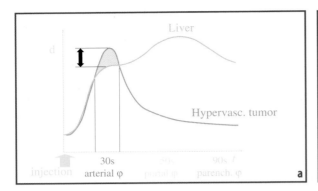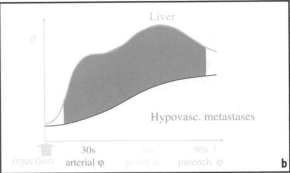

Fig. 1a, b. Enhancement profiles of normal liver and liver tumors during the three vascular phases of contrast-enhanced CT. The vascular phases are defined in relation to the moment of injection (time 0), and are the arterial phase (20–35 s), portal venous phase (50–60 s), and late (parenchymal) phase (after several minutes). **a** Normal liver and typical hypervascular tumor (e.g., focal nodular hyperplasia, adenoma). **b** Normal liver and typical hypovascular tumor (e.g., hypovascular metastasis) (Reproduced from [21], with permission)

to the moment when the hypervascular lesions are most conspicuous, in order to obtain the most diagnostic information.

One advantage of MDCT over single-slice helical CT is that acquisition of images is faster. Thus, with MDCT it is possible to scan the entire liver during the brief late arterial phase. This should improve our ability to explore the liver for hypervascular lesions, which are hyperintense to normal liver tissue during this phase, but will not have a major impact on the detection of hypovascular lesions. Nonetheless, the increased resolution of MDCT afforded by thinner slices should also improve the detection of small hypovascular nodules.

Several studies have now clearly shown that the ability to detect lesions at contrast-enhanced MDCT depends on the parameters of contrast medium injection, especially the concentration and volume of contrast medium and the injection rate [3-6]. The best visualization of hypervascular tumors is obtained during the arterial phase with the use of highly concentrated contrast media (small volume) and high injection rate. Enhancement of liv-

er tissue during the portal phase depends mostly on the total dose of contrast medium.

Another advantage of MDCT is the ability to reduce the effective slice thickness without requiring a longer scan duration or a shorter scan length [7]. Slice thickness varies with acquisition parameters such as collimation, table feed per rotation, and pitch; depending on the scanner model and on the protocols for multislice data interpolation and reconstruction, a defined selection of slice thicknesses is available. However, multiple data sets with different slice thicknesses may be reconstructed from the same raw data with the only requirement that the slice thicknesses be larger than or equal to the collimation. The choice of slice thickness for the reconstructed data sets, dictated by the clinical situation, involves a compromise between spatial resolution (which is improved with thin slices) and image noise (which is disproportionately high when the slice thickness is chosen to equal the collimation).

The typical MDCT protocol (Table 1) starts with a bolus injection of iodinated contrast medi-

Table 1. Typical parameters for MDCT of the liver

X-ray generation	
Kilovolt	120 kV
Effective current	160 mA
Scan parameters	
Rotation time	0.5 s
Collimation	2.5 mm
Table feed per rotation	12.5 mm
Slice thickness	5 mm
Increment	3 mm
Contrast medium administration	
Iodine concentration	400 mg/ml
Volume	1.7–2.0 ml/kg body weight
Flow rate	4 ml/s

um at a flow rate of 4 ml/s. The slice thickness is commonly 5 mm. For hypervascular lesions (both benign tumors and hypervascular metastases), a dual-phase acquisition is performed. First, the liver is imaged during the late arterial phase 35 s after injection; use of a bolus-triggering system is advantageous for precise timing. Then, imaging is performed during the portal phase, 60 s after injection, with the same scanning parameters. When appropriate, imaging is also performed in the late phase, after 3 min. Alternatively, for hypovascular metastases, a single acquisition 60 s after the administration of contrast medium is often sufficient.

Diagnosis of Benign Liver Tumors

Benign tumors are often discovered incidentally when patients undergo imaging examinations for other reasons. Hemangioma, the most frequently encountered benign liver tumor, has a prevalence of 2%–20% in the general population. Focal nodular hyperplasia (FNH) is the second most common benign tumor, but its prevalence is much lower than that of hemangioma. While adenoma of the liver ranks third in prevalence among benign tumors, it is rare. Nonetheless, it is important to clearly distinguish adenoma from the more common benign tumors because adenoma poses a risk of rupture and thus requires surgical excision, while hemangioma and FNH can be managed conservatively. Furthermore, since adenoma may be confused with malignant hepatocellular carcinoma, a tissue specimen must be obtained for a confident histopathological diagnosis.

When a benign tumor is suspected on the basis of a previous imaging examination, further imaging is usually performed to confirm its benign nature and to rule out malignancy. However, differentiating some malignant and benign tumors is

difficult, especially in the case of adenoma. A practical first approach consists of trying to confidently diagnose those benign tumors that can be managed conservatively. In fact, 90% of benign liver tumors are hemangiomas or FNHs, which do not require surgical treatment. If a highly specific imaging protocol can provide an unequivocal diagnosis of these lesions, the patient does not need to undergo surgery. Thus, when a benign liver tumor is suspected, the imaging strategy can be simplified to obtaining a confident diagnosis of hemangioma or FNH. This strategy resolves over 90% of cases of benign liver tumors.

Hemangiomas

Most cavernous hemangiomas are easily diagnosed on the basis of their characteristic imaging appearance (Fig. 2): on unenhanced CT images, they have an attenuation value near that of blood; after the bolus administration of contrast medium, they exhibit globular or nodular peripheral enhancement, again with attentuation similar to that of blood; finally, during the late imaging phase, they appear opaque. This typical presentation has been seen with monodetector CT for many years, and multidetector technology does not seem to provide additional diagnostic information. Nonetheless, some hemangiomas present atypical characteristics and may be confused with other lesions, resulting in a misdiagnosis [8]. Atypical enhancement at CT is observed in cases of large heterogeneous hemangiomas with incomplete late filling, in hyalinized hemangiomas without peripheral enhancement, and in cystic hemangiomas, small hemangiomas, and hemangiomas with adjacent arterioportal shunts. With the exception of small hemangiomas, the atypical appearances are caused by lesion characteristics that can-

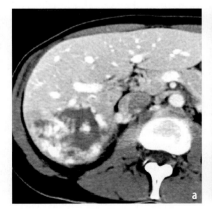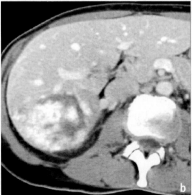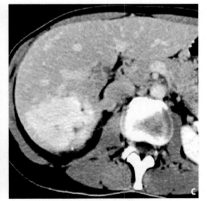

Fig. 2a-c. Typical CT appearance of hemangioma. **a** The arterial-phase CT image reveals globular enhancement with attenuation similar to that of blood. **b** The portal-phase image shows the progressive filling of the tumor. **c** Persistent opacification is seen in the late vascular phase (Reproduced from [21], with permission)

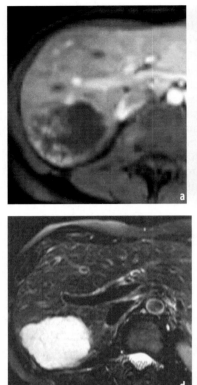
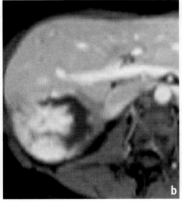
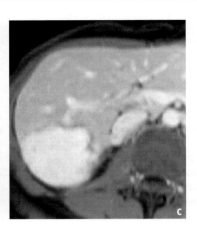
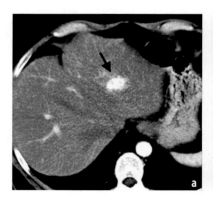

Fig. 3a-d. Typical appearance of a hemangioma at MRI. The tumor is the same as that shown in Fig. 2. The enhancement pattern seen at MRI is similar to that observed with CT. **a-c** T1-weighted MR images. **a** Arterial phase image after contrast medium administration. **b** Portal-phase image. **c** Late-phase image. **d** Contrast-enhanced T2-weighted MR image reveals marked hyperintensity of the lesion (Reproduced from [21], with permission)

not be visualized in the arterial phase; therefore, it is unlikely that MDCT will prove advantageous in these situations. Moreover, most atypical hemangiomas can be readily diagnosed at magnetic resonance imaging (MRI) on the basis of the relatively strong hyperintensity on T2-weighted images. Since the sensitivity and specificity of MRI in detecting atypical hemangiomas are greater than 90%, CT does not play a big role in the diagnosis of these lesions (Fig. 3).

The diagnosis of small hemangiomas may be improved with the use of multiphase CT. The atypical enhancement pattern of these benign tumors consists in a homogeneous, rapid filling with contrast agent during the arterial phase (Figs. 4, 5), rather than the usual early globular enhancement and opacification in the late phase. Kim et al. [9] assessed the accuracy of three-phase helical CT in differentiating 37 small hemangiomas from 49 other small hypervascular malignancies in 86 patients. The authors confirmed the atypical enhancement pattern of small hemangiomas. They also reported that the specificity of the technique for the differentiation of small hemangiomas from malignant lesions was as high as 95% when the lesions had the same attenuation as the blood pool in the combined nonenhanced, arterial and portal phases.

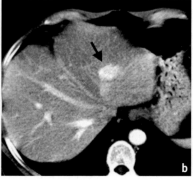

Fig. 4a, b. Small hemangioma with atypical appearance at CT (*arrows*). **a** The arterial-phase image reveals a global enhancement of the hemangioma. Because of tumor size, progressive filling is not present. **b** The portal-phase image shows persistant hyperattenuation. Because of this atypical presentation, it is often difficult to distinguish small hemangiomas from other hypervascular tumors (Reproduced from [21], with permission)

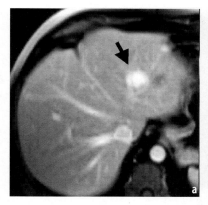
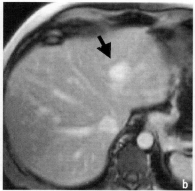
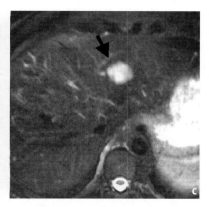

Fig. 5a-c. Small hemangioma with atypical appearance at MRI (*arrows*). The tumor is the same as that shown in Figure 4. **a, b** T1-weighted MR images reveal global enhancement during the arterial phase (**a**) and portal phase (**b**) similarly to CT. **c** T2-weighted image shows that the lesion is typically hyperintense relative to normal liver tissue, confirming the diagnosis of hemangioma (Reproduced from [21], with permission)

Focal Nodular Hyperplasia

Although FNH is a rare tumor, its incidence is increasing as a result of the improved diagnostic capabilities offered by modern cross-sectional imaging techniques. FNH probably results from a hyperplastic response to a local vascular abnormality. Since these benign lesions contain normal hepatocytes, needle biopsy is unlikely to be diagnostic and imaging is necessary to make a specific diagnosis.

The appearance of FNH at CT is well described [10, 11]. These lesions are usually homogeneous and isoattenuating to the normal liver on baseline CT images. After the administration of contrast medium, FNHs typically exhibit homogeneous bright enhancement and a hypoattenuating central scar in the late arterial phase (Fig. 6). Radiating hypointense fibrous bands and septa arising from the central scar are less frequently observed but are also characteristic of FNH. During the portal phase, the attenuation returns to that of normal liver, making the lesions difficult to detect. In the late vascular phase, the central scar and septa are often hyperattenuating due to their fibrotic contents. Dilated feeding arteries penetrating the central scar and draining veins running along the surface of the lesion may be seen in large FNH. Additional common features of FNH are a homogeneous enhancement pattern except for the scar area, well-defined margins, lack of capsule and lobulated contours.

The diagnosis of FNH is definitive when all the common imaging features are present. Since the most reliable appearance of FNH is the hyperattenuation relative to normal liver tissue in the arterial phase, the use of MDCT could be advantageous for rapidly surveying the entire liver for FNH. However, the current imaging modality of choice for detecting FNH is MRI. On noncontrasted T2-weighted MR images, FNHs are isointense to normal liver with the exception of the central scar which is hyperintense (Fig. 7). On contrast-enhanced MR images, FNHs have the same imaging characteristics as they do on contrast-enhanced CT. Thus, MRI is preferred to CT for these lesions since it does not imply an exposure to iodinated contrast agent nor to irradiation.

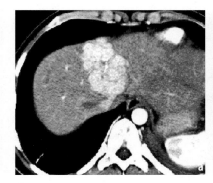
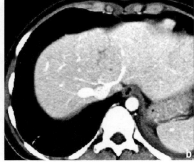
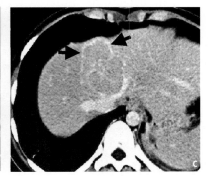

Fig. 6a-c. Typical appearance of focal nodular nyperplasia (FNH) at contrast-enhanced CT. **a** The late arterial-phase image reveals a lesion with homogeneous bright enhancement and a hypoattenuating central scar containing feeding arteries. **b** On the portal-phase image, the lesion is isoattenuating to normal liver tissue while the central scar is hypoattenuating. **c** At delayed-phase imaging, the central scar becomes hyperattenuating and the draining peripheral veins are visible (*arrows*) (Reproduced from [21], with permission)

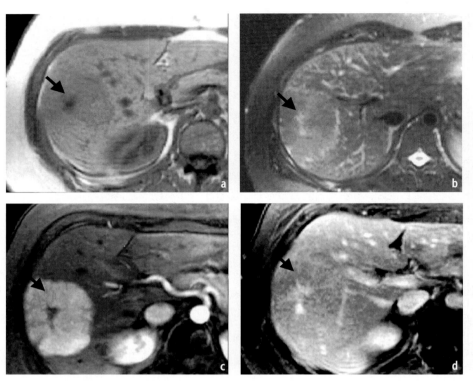

Fig. 7a-d. Typical appearance of FNH at MRI. **a, b** The tumor mass is homogeneously isointense to normal liver on T1-weighted (**a**) and T2-weighted (**b**) non-contrasted images. The central scar (*arrow*) is hypointense on the T1-weighted image and hyperintense on the T2-weighted image. **c, d** With contrast-enhanced MRI, the tumor exhibits homogeneous hyperintensity during the arterial phase of T1-weighted imaging (**c**); during the portal phase the tumor mass becomes isointense while the central scar (*arrow*) is hyperintense (**d**) (Reproduced from [21], with permission)

The diagnosis of FNH is more difficult when atypical imaging features are observed. Almost 50% of FNHs are considered atypical, and these fall into two main groups.

- One subset of atypical FNH lacks the central scar, while all other usual imaging characteristics are present. A central scar may be missing in small FNHs or in very large FNH when the scar is thin, near the surface of the tumor, or simply absent. The differential diagnosis of these atypical FNHs includes all hypervascular tumors, including adenomas and hepatocellular carcinomas. The diagnosis is confirmed with MRI, which may often reveal the thin central scar not seen on CT. It is also easier to demonstrate the homogeneity of the tumor and the isointensity to normal liver with MRI than with CT (Figs. 8, 9). The use of liver-specific MR contrast agents may better delineate the central scar [12]. Finally, large-needle percutaneous biopsy permits a histopathological diagnosis when radiological features are non-specific but compatible with the diagnosis of FNH; the use of biopsy in addition to imaging techniques resulted in a confident diagnosis of FNH in over 90% of cases and avoided unnecessary surgery [13].

- A second atypical presentation of FNH consists of pseudocapsule or inhomogeneous content due to focal telangiectatic areas, fat deposits, or necrosis. A confident diagnosis is almost impossible to make on the basis of imaging results, and the tumor should be surgically resected.

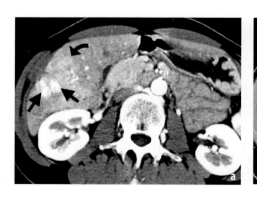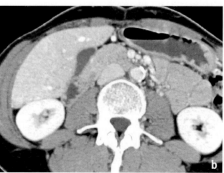

Fig. 8a, b. Atypical appearance of FNH at contrast-enhanced CT. **a** On the arterial-phase image, the tumor (*straight arrows*) appears hypervascular; a pseudocapule is seen while the central scar is not depicted. In addition, there is abnormal peritumoral arterial perfusion (*curved arrow*). **b** In the portal phase, the tumor is no longer visible (Reproduced from [21], with permission)

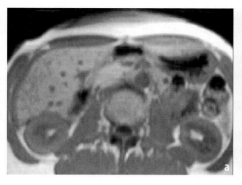
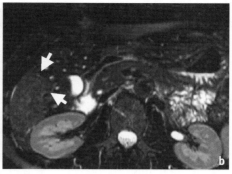

Fig. 9a, b. Atypical appearance of FNH at MRI. The tumor is the same as that shown in Figure 8. **a** Uncontrasted T1-weighted image. **b** T2-weighted image. The lesion is quite undetectable, because it is almost isointense to normal liver tissue. The lesion is therefore most likely FNH although the central scar is not detectable; a diagnosis is only possible with percutaneous biopsy (Reproduced from [21], with permission)

Liver Adenoma

Like FNH, adenoma also typically presents as a hyperattenuating area on contrast-enhanced CT during the late arterial phase. Ruppert-Kohlmayr et al. [14] found that differences in attenuation value during the arterial phase of helical CT, but not during the unenhanced and portal venous phases, could distinguish 45 FNHs from 18 hepatocellular adenomas. During the arterial phase, the mean attenuation value of FNH was significantly higher than that of adenoma. An enhancement threshold value of 1.6 correctly distinguished FNHs from adenomas (all FNHs were positioned above and

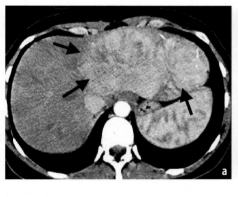
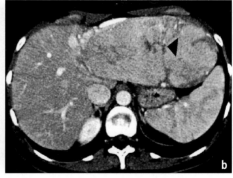

Fig. 10a, b. Liver adenoma imaged with contrast-enhanced CT. The tumor (*arrows*) is moderately hypervascular and is heterogeneous during the late arterial (**a**) and portal (**b**) phases. A false image of central scar is visible (*arrowhead*) (Reproduced from [21], with permission)

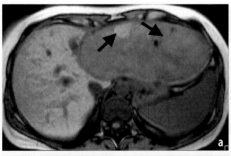
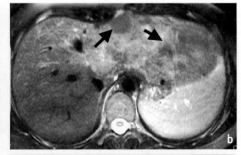
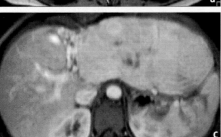
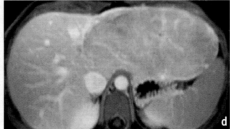

Fig. 11a-d. Liver adenoma imaged with MRI. The tumor is the same as that shown in Fig. 10. **a** Uncontrasted T1-weighted image. **b** T2-weighted image. Both images show an inhomogeneous tumor with nodular pattern (*arrows*) that precludes the diagnosis of FNH. **c, d** T1-weighted images after gadolinium injection reveal slight heterogeneous enhancement in the arterial phase, while during the portal phase the tumor mass becomes isointense (Reproduced from [21], with permission)

87% of adenomas were positioned below this enhancement value); the accuracy of this approach was 96%. The clinical usefulness of these promising results is, however, limited since they do not refer to small tumors. Moreover, most large adenomas can be distinguished from FNH when they contain a fibrotic capsule, subcapsular feeding arteries, and necrotic or fatty areas (Figs. 10, 11).

The imaging appearance of adenoma is often similar to that of a hepatocellular carcinoma developing in an otherwise healthy liver. Therefore, the final diagnosis of adenoma cannot be made with imaging alone, and suspected adenomas must be surgically removed.

Diagnosis of Liver Metastases

When a patient is diagnosed with a non-hepatic primary malignancy, both the initial therapeutic approach and the subsequent management are conditioned by the results of a liver survey for metastases. In such cases, the liver survey is usually performed using CT. If liver metastases are found, CT is then used to determine the number of lesions and to characterize them for size and location. On this basis, treatment with resection or percutaneous radiofrequency ablation may be considered, and chemotherapy regimens are tailored according to lesion size.

The characteristics of an ideal imaging modality to screen for liver metastases [15] include:

- High negative predictive value, to confidently rule out metastatic disease in patients apparently free of liver lesions,
- High sensitivity, to detect small metastases distant from lesions that can otherwise be treated by resection, and
- Minimal invasiveness, since these patients require numerous imaging examinations during the course of the disease

Depending on the type of primary tumor, a liver metastasis can be hypervascular or hypovascular compared to normal liver tissue; this main characteristic determines the choice of imaging protocol.

Hypervascular Metastases

Liver metastases tend to be hypervascular in cases of primary tumors of the thyroid or pancreatic islet cells, carcinoid tumors, renal cell carcinoma, some breast tumors and melanoma. These tumors are best detected during the late arterial phase on contrast-enhanced CT, when they are hyperattenuating relative to the surrounding liver tissue. Although MDCT has not yet been investigated as a technique for diagnosing hypervascular metastases, the arterial phase of helical CT was effective in detecting carcinoid liver metastases [16].

Hypovascular Metastases

The majority of liver metastases is hypovascular, and develop from primary tumors of the colon and rectum (most frequent), pancreas, lung, urothelium, prostate, and from gynecological malignancies (except choriocarcinoma). At CT, these metastases are hypoattenuating during the arterial and portal phases. Thin peripheral enhancement, necrosis, and calcification may also be seen, depending on the type of primary tumor. Hypovascular metastases are best detected during the portal phase, when the difference in attenuation between lesion and normal tissue is greatest. Therefore, the timing of imaging for hypovascular lesions is less crucial than that required for hypervascular lesions which are best detected in the brief arterial phase.

Currently, hypovascular metastases are efficiently diagnosed with helical CT. Valls et al. [17] used single-detector helical CT to prospectively screen 157 patients with hepatic metastases. Helical CT detected 247 of 290 liver metastases for an overall detection rate of 85%; the false-positive rate was 4%. It is unlikely that MDCT will improve these results overall, but the systematic use of thin slices and the high resolution of MDCT may augment the detection of small metastases (Fig. 12). In fact, the false-negative findings of Valls et al. [17] were all due to lesions smaller than 1 cm.

The advantage of the thin collimation of MDCT for detecting small hypoattenuating lesions was studied by Haider et al. [18]: when 88 lesions smaller than or equal to 1.5 cm were imaged at two different collimation widths, the sensitivity for lesion detection was significantly better at 2.5 mm (82%) than at 5.0 mm (66%). However, when only metastatic lesions were considered, the sensitivities for detection were 80% for both collimation values [18]. These results raise two important issues:

- First, with the same contrast medium injection parameters and scan timing, thinner collimation did not improve the detection of small liver metastases. This finding may be due to increased image noise or failure to improve tumor conspicuousness. The most important determinant of the conspicuousness of small tumors is considered to be the dose of iodinated contrast agent, as illustrated by the high sensitivity of CT during arterial portography [19].
- Second, thinner collimation did improve the

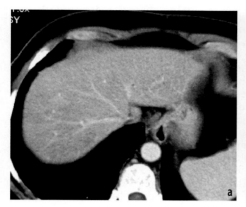 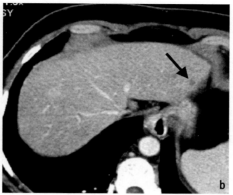

Fig. 12a, b. Small liver metastasis derived from a primary tumor of the colon. Images were obtained with MDCT. **a** Image obtained with 8-mm slice thickness; the lesion is not detected. **b** Image obtained with 5-mm slice thickness; a hypoattenuating lesion is seen (*arrow*). The smaller slice thickness is necessary to detect small hypoattenuating lesions

detection of small hypoattenuating lesions unrelated to metastatic disease. This issue has been more recently investigated by Jang et al. [20], who retrospectively reviewed the results of preoperative single-phase helical CT performed on 1,133 patients with known gastric or colorectal cancer; with this technique, 881 small (≤1.5 cm) hypoattenuating lesions were found in 268 patients. A final diagnosis of benignity was made for 693 lesions (78%) while 188 lesions (21%) were determined to be metastatic. The prevalence of small hypoattenuating lesions (25.5%) determined with helical CT was greater than that obtained with conventional CT, while metastases presenting as small hypoattenuating lesions were rare (2%). These results confirm that the increase in number of hypoattenuating lesions observed with recent CT techniques is attributable to improved visibility of small benign tumors rather than better detection of small metastases. From a clinical point of view, detecting more metastases but also more benign lesions easily confused with small metastases is not useful, unless a differential diagnosis is possible. Most of these small benign tumors were cystic lesions including biliary hamartomas and focal fatty sparing.

Jang et al. [20] suggested that the differential diagnosis between true metastases and cysts (based on water attenuation and sharp margins) or fatty infiltration (angular margins and typical location) is possible with careful analysis of CT findings.

On the basis of the current evidence, the use of collimation of less than 5 mm for the diagnosis of small metastases is questionable. One imaging strategy could involve the use of thin-collimation MDCT to detect lesions followed by MRI to characterize them, especially since small cysts are better demonstrated on T2-weighted MR images (Fig. 13) and focal fatty infiltration is well detected on T1-weighted MR sequences.

Conclusions

The advantages of MDCT include a reduced image acquisition time, easier timing of scanning in synchronization with liver vascular phases, and better spatial resolution (from the systematic use of 5-mm slices). The reduced acquisition time allows more images to be obtained within one breath hold. In clinical practice, these technical advances

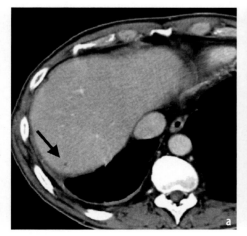 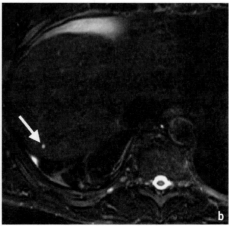

Fig. 13a, b. False small metastasis in the right lobe of the liver, detected during preoperative imaging examination for a colon cancer metastasis in the left lobe (*not shown*). **a** The possible small metastasis is hypoattenuating as depicted on contrast-enhanced MDCT (*arrow*). **b** It is hyperintense on the T2-weighted MR image (*arrow*), suggesting a cystic nature. At surgery, the lesion was found to be a biliary hamartoma

result in high-quality CT images and improved reproducibility. However, they have not yet translated into improvements in the diagnosis of benign and metastatic liver tumors, so that no significant changes in the diagnostic approaches may be advanced at the present time. MRI remains the gold standard examination for the investigation of suspected benign liver tumors, and it is unlikely that future technical refinements of the MDCT technique will change this. CT is nonetheless an important technique for the detection of hepatic metastases. Whether thinner collimation, more concentrated contrast medium, post-bolus saline "pushes", or other innovative protocols for contrast medium administration will improve the detection of liver metastases with CT remains the topic of future investigations.

References

1. Spielman A, Nelson R (2003) Liver. In: Bonomo L, Foley DW, Imhof H, Rubin G (eds) Multidetector CT technology: advances in imaging techniques. Royal Society of Medicine, London, pp 129-139
2. Foley WD, Mallisee TA, Hohenwalter MD (2000) Multiphase hepatic CT with multirow detector CT scanners. AJR Am J Roentgenol 175:679-685
3. Berland LL, Lee JY (1998) Comparison of contrast media injection rates and volumes for hepatic dynamic incremented CT. Invest Radiol 23:918-922
4. Awai K, Takada K, Onishi H et al (2002) Aortic and hepatic enhancement and tumor-to-liver contrast, analysis of the effect of different concentrations of contast material at multi-detector row helical CT. Radiology 224:757-763
5. Fleischmann D (2003) Use of high-concentration contrast media: principles and rationale – vascular district. In: Bonomo L, Foley DW, Imhof H, Rubin G (eds) Multidetector CT technology: advances in imaging techniques. Royal Society of Medicine, London, pp 27-38
6. Brink JA (2003) Use of high-concentration contrast media (HCCM): principles and rationale – body CT. Eur J Radiol 45[Suppl 1]:S53-S58
7. Prokop M (2003) General principles of MDCT. Eur J Radiol 45[Suppl 1]:S4-S10
8. Vilgrain V, Boulos L, Vullierme MP et al (2000) Imaging of atypical hemangiomas of the liver with pathologic correlation. Radiographics 20:379-397
9. Kim T, Federle MP, Baron RL et al (2001) Discrimination of small hemangiomas from hypervascular malignant tumors smaller than 3 cm with three-phase helical CT. Radiology 219:699-706
10. Van Beers B, Horsmans Y, Sempoux C (2003) Scanner multidétecteur face à l'IRM dans les tumeurs bénignes du foie. J Radiol 84:445-456
11. Brancatelli G, Federle MP, Grazioli L et al (2001) Focal nodular hyperplasia: CT findings with emphasis on multiphasic helical CT in 78 patients. Radiology 219:61-68
12. Ba-Ssalamah A, Schima W, Schmook MT et al (2002) Atypical focal nodular hyperplasia of the liver: imaging features of nonspecific and liver-specific MR contrast agents. AJR Am J Roentgenol 179:1447-1456
13. Fabre M, Neyra M (1995) Role of fine needle puncture in the diagnosis of a hepatic mass. Ann Pathol 15:380-387 [article in French]
14. Ruppert-Kohlmayr A, Uggowitzer M, Kugler C et al (2001) Focal nodular hyperplasia and hepatocellular adenoma of the liver: differentiation with multiphasic helical CT. AJR Am J Roentgenol 176:1493-1498
15. Vilgrain V (2003) Scanner multidétecteur face à l'IRM dans les tumeurs malignes du foie. J Radiol 84:459-470
16. Paulson EK, McDermott VG, Keogan MT et al (1998) Carcinoid metastases to the liver: role of triple-phase helical CT. Radiology 206:143-150
17. Valls C, Andia E, Sanchez A et al (2001) Hepatic metastases from colorectal cancer: preoperative detection and assessment of resectability with helical CT. Radiology 218:55-60
18. Haider MA, Amitai MM, Rappaport DC et al (2002) Multi-detector row helical CT in preoperative assessment of small (<1.5 cm) liver metastases: is thinner collimation better? Radiology 225:137-142
19. Kehagias D, Metafa A, Hatziioannou A et al (2000) Comparison of CT, MRI and CT during arterial portography in the detection of malignant hepatic lesions. Hepatogastroenterology 47:1399-1403
20. Jag HJ, Lim HK, Lee AJ et al (2002) Small hypoattenuating lesions in the liver on single-phase helical CT in preoperative patients with gastric and colorectal cancer: prevalence, significance and differentiating features. J Comput Assist Tomogr 26(5):718-724
21. Valette PJ, Pilleul F, Crombé-Ternamian A (2003) MDCT of Benign Liver tumors and metastases. In: Eur Radiol Vol 13 [Suppl. 3]:M31-M41

II.2

MDCT of Primary Liver Malignancy

Alfonso Marchianò

Introduction

In daily practice, common indications for abdominal computed tomography (CT) include detection of liver malignancies, characterization of liver lesions suggested by other imaging tests, and evaluation of chronic liver diseases. Hepatocellular carcinoma (HCC) is the most common primary malignant hepatic neoplasm and its incidence is increasing. HCC accounts for 6% of all human cancers worldwide, being the fifth most common malignancy in men and the tenth in women [1]. HCC usually occurs as a complication of chronic liver disease and most often arises in patients with hepatic cirrhosis. Imaging the cirrhotic liver is a technical challenge for CT. Cirrhosis alters the normal parenchyma with various degenerative processes such as fibrosis, scarring, and nodular regeneration. Not only are these tumors difficult to detect in patients with cirrhosis, but the alterations inherent in cirrhosis create lesions that may simulate a tumor. Most HCCs are hypervascular lesions that typically enhance during the phase of maximum hepatic arterial enhancement. Therefore, such lesions have often been difficult to detect with conventional CT of the liver, in which only portal venous-phase imaging was performed because of the long scanning time.

During the past decade, the introduction of helical CT technology has opened the door to new approaches to liver imaging. With its short acquisition time, spiral CT allows imaging of the entire liver twice, before equilibrium: a hepatic arterial dominant phase and a portal venous phase of enhancement [2]. Several studies have demonstrated that this biphasic approach to scanning greatly improves the detection of HCC (Fig. 1). Because of the vascular nature of these lesions, there is evidence that a greater number of HCC nodules are detected when images are acquired with dual-phase CT compared with portal venous phase imaging alone [3, 4].

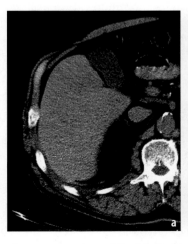 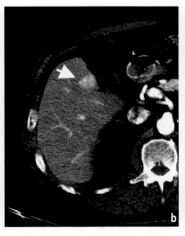 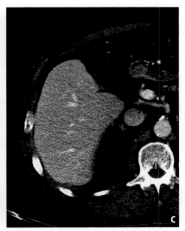

Fig. 1a-c. Unenhanced CT of the liver in a patient with cirrhosis: no lesion is seen. (**a**) During the arterial phase a hypervascular hepatocellular carcinoma (HCC) is well depicted (*arrow* in **b**). The portal venous phase (**c**) missed the lesion

Table 1. Protocols for liver MDCT

Number of detector rows	4	16
Detector configuration (mm)	4×2.5	16×0.75
kV/effective mA/rotation time	140/200/0.5	140/200/0.5
Pitch	1.5	1.75
Reconstruction thickness (mm)		
Axial	5	5
3D/MPR	2.5	0.75
IV contrast volume	100 ml/30 ml	100 ml/ 30 ml
(400 mg I/ml saline)		
Injection rate	4 ml/s	4 ml/s
Scan/delay (s)	35 s/55 s	35 s/55 s
MPR = multiplanar reformations		

Dual-phase CT has become the most common screening tool for depicting HCC, including screening the population at risk, confirming the diagnosis, planning treatment, and follow-up after treatment. Magnetic resonance imaging is used primarily to evaluate liver lesions with indeterminate findings on CT and to image patients with a contraindication for iodinated contrast material.

Multidetector row-CT (MDCT) offers considerable advantages, which include improved temporal resolution, improved spatial resolution in the z-axis, and larger anatomical coverage. As a result we can scan the abdomen within reasonable breath-hold times, with decreased respiratory and motion artifacts and higher image quality. With the improvement in technology, optimization of the scanning techniques is needed to maximize the benefit of new imaging capabilities.

MDCT Parameters

Scanning protocols for liver MDCT are characterized by a combination of thin slices and high pitches. The use of the fastest gantry rotation speed (0.4–0.5 s) is advantageous, with the exception of patients with a large habitus, who could require a slower gantry rotation speed in order to achieve adequate image quality. Typical scanning protocols for liver MDCT are shown in Table 1.

High spatial resolution along the z-axis with nearly isotropic voxels reduces volume averaging effects and is the basis for multiplanar reformations of high quality. Coronal and sagittal reformations are very helpful for planning of surgery and for the localization of lesions in relation to the liver segments (Fig. 2).

The excellent quality of the three-dimensional data sets obtained with thin collimation improves the quality of CT angiography (CTA) [5] of the liver and mesenteric vessels. This technique can be important in patients that are candidates for hepatic resection, liver transplantation, or transarterial chemoembolization. In this respect, CT porto-angiography is probably superior to classic angiography. CTA can provide a complete picture of the complex collaterization of the portal vein in potential liver transplantation recipients (Fig. 3).

Axial images can be prospectively reconstructed thicker than the collimation used during the data acquisition in order to reduce image noise. Indeed, thinner slices have a major impact on radiologist productivity and operating costs (film printing or Picture Archiving Communication System, PACS) and there is some evidence that the routine use of a slice thickness of less than 5 mm does not improve the sensitivity of CT for detecting small HCC in patients with cirrhosis [6].

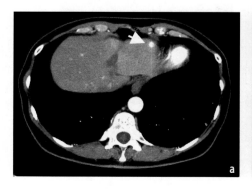 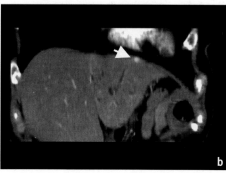

Fig. 2a, b. Hepatic MDCT. **a** A hypervascular lesion (*arrow*) in the dome of the liver is seen in the late arterial phase. **b** Coronal multiplanar reformation (MPR) allows a better anatomical delineation of this subcapsular lesion

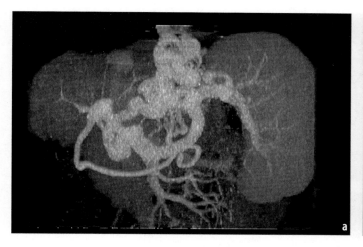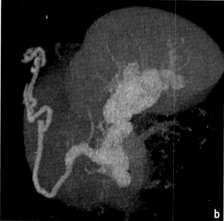

Fig. 3a, b. Severe portal hypertension in a cirrhotic patient. Anterior (**a**) and right lateral maximum intensity projection (**b**) images show a recanalized paraumbilical vein and large left gastric and esophageal varix that drains the portal vein circulation

Scan Protocols

Foley and Mallisee [7] proposed a triple-pass technique with MDCT for the detection of hypervascular neoplasms. The ability to scan through the entire liver in 10 s or less allows the acquisition of two separate sets of CT images of the liver within the time generally regarded as the hepatic arterial dominant phase in single-slice CT. Early and late arterial-phase images can be acquired during the hepatic arterial dominant phase within a single breath hold. The first acquisition provides a true arterial phase with no admixture of enhanced portal venous blood, whereas in the late arterial phase an initial opacification of the portal venous blood occurs (portal venous inflow phase). The third pass, acquired with a delay of 60 s after the start of infusion of contrast material, corresponds to the portal venous phase of the conventional biphasic protocol used with a single-detector scanner.

Foley and Mallisee [7] concluded that, although hypervascular lesions are best detected during the late arterial phase, early arterial-phase images were useful for providing a volume data set for CT arteriography of the hepatic and mesenteric arterial road map. Murakami et al. [8] reported a slight advantage of the early arterial phase in terms of the detection rate of lesions. Therefore the authors found a distinct benefit in the combined analysis of the early and later arterial-phase images for the recognition of the so-called pseudolesions, an important problem of cirrhotic liver imaging.

A large number of benign lesions that simulate HCC can be encountered in patients with cirrhosis; these include arterial-portal venous shunts, focal confluent fibrosis, transient hepatic attenuation difference, and flash filling hemangiomas. In two more-recent papers, double arterial-phase CT showed no significant improvement compared with single arterial-phase CT alone for detecting hypervascular HCC [9, 10]. Therefore the role of double arterial-phase CT remains controversial and it is not yet routinely included in CT protocols.

In clinical practice the acquisition of an additional late image, during the equilibrium phase, is considered optional, although it can help to better characterize indeterminate hepatic lesions. This phase begins approximately 90–120 s after initiation of bolus injection. During this phase the difference in concentration of the iodinated contrast agent between the intravascular and the extravascular extracellular space is progressively reduced. Hence a large proportion of liver tumors tend to disappear during this phase. Nevertheless, delayed contrast-enhanced CT can improve the detection of cholangiocarcinoma. This is probably related to the larger extracellular diffusion space in the fibrous tumoral stroma [11]. Delayed peripheral enhancement of cholangiocarcinoma and "filling-in" patterns of hemangioma are well known signs in the differential diagnosis of hepatic masses (Fig. 4).

Finally some well-differentiated HCCs, which have a normal or only slightly increased arterial supply but a decreased portal supply, are only visible on delayed-phase images [12] as low-attenuation nodules.

Contrast Medium

One of the major advantages of MDCT over standard helical CT is that it takes significantly less time to scan a target organ and we can obtain better differentiation of arterial and portal venous perfusion phases. Frederick et al. [13] postulated that the time window for the hepatic arterial dom-

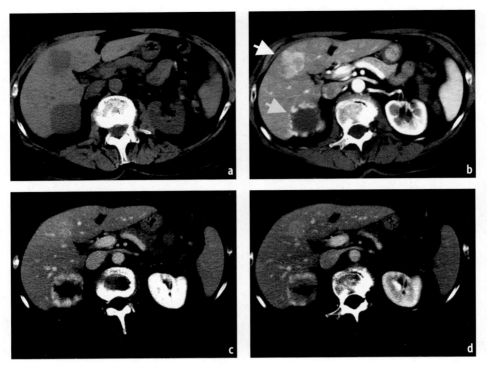

Fig. 4a-d. Hepatic MDCT with acquisitions in different enhancement phases . Two distinctive hepatic lesions are clearly depicted. A typical hemangioma with a globular enhancement and a progressive and persistent opacification (*yellow arrow*) and a malignant hypervascular lesion, barely hyperdense in the portal venous and delayed phases (cholangiocarcinoma) (*white arrow*)

inant phase is too brief to image properly using conventional helical CT technology. With scan times in the range of 10 s, pure arterial phase imaging without venous overlay can be achieved. With the evolution of MDCT, the time required to scan the liver is further reduced. However, the schemes of contrast medium administration need to be revised with regard to the optimal timing, total volume, rate of administration, and the ideal iodine concentration.

Ideal imaging of the hepatic arterial phase requires the scan delay to be optimized. A number of techniques are available to achieve this, including a fixed time delay, a test bolus, and automated scanning technology. At many institutions, CT is performed with the same empirically determined delay. This occasionally leads to incorrect timing

(Fig. 5), as with short acquisition times one may completely miss the bolus if the delay is not properly chosen. For dedicated liver imaging, a test bolus injection or automatic bolus triggering is strongly recommended. The test bolus is accurate, but it does need an additional 12–20 ml of contrast material and time to be performed. The computer-assisted bolus-tracking techniques offered by different CT manufacturers provide major advantages, including automatic initiation of the scan once a contrast threshold is reached.

The recommended dose of iodine to be injected ranges between 40 and 45 g. Although in hepatic imaging a good arterial phase can be obtained at a lower dose, the total dose should not be reduced, since the principal determinant of parenchymal enhancement is the total iodine dose.

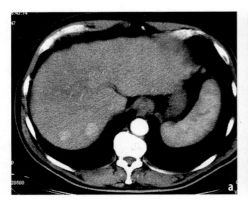

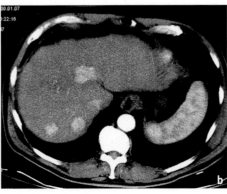

Fig. 5a, b. Axial CT scans during the arterial dominant phase performed in two different sessions in the same patient. The same contrast medium protocol was used in both, but a different delay was chosen. With an incorrect delay, scan lesion conspicuity is significantly decreased: compare (**a**) to (**b**)

With shorter scan time windows, it is absolutely critical to increase the arterial enhancement more rapidly. The main injection parameter influencing arterial enhancement is iodine flux (milligrams of iodine per second). Two injection parameters can be adjusted to increase arterial enhancement: the flow rate and the concentration of the contrast medium.

In dual-phase CT, a high flow rate of at least 4–5 ml/s is recommended. Although hepatic enhancement is relatively insensitive to flow rate (because it is essentially correlated with the total amount of iodine used), a higher flow rate guarantees an earlier as well as a greater peak arterial enhancement. Therefore a high flow rate improves the temporal separation of arterial and portal phases [14].

The rates at which contrast media are administered have increased significantly over the past few years and there is no doubt that this trend will continue when shorter scan time windows become available. High infusion rates, however, are limited by the quality of the intravenous access and greater attention must be paid to the inherent risks of contrast medium extravasation [15].

A higher concentration of contrast medium is an effective alternative. Several data in the literature support the hypothesis that an increase in contrast medium concentration results in a greater degree of enhancement and diagnostic efficacy for hypervascular lesions. Several studies include the comparison of different concentrations of contrast

agents, with the same volume of contrast or the same total iodine dose. Hanninen et al. [16] compared two different protocols of biphasic liver imaging with Iopromide at two different iodine concentrations (300 mg/ml vs. 370 mg/ml) adopting the same delivery rate and scan delay time. In patients with HCC, a significantly higher contrast enhancement of the lesions was observed. However, since a fixed volume (180 ml) was chosen, a larger amount of iodine was administered with the more concentrated contrast medium. In a more recent report, Awai et al. [17] compared two iodine concentrations of Iopamidol (300 mg/ml and 370 mg/ml) with the same total iodine load per patient per kilogram body weight. A triple-pass MDCT technique was used in patients with HCC. During the first arterial phase the attenuation differences between the hepatic tumors and the hepatic parenchyma were significantly higher with the more concentrated contrast medium.

In both reports there was no significant difference in the mean hepatic enhancement between the two different concentrations during the arterial phase. This finding is not unexpected since during the arterial dominant phase the liver parenchyma receives only a small amount of contrast material, compared with the majority of the hypervascular HCCs. Therefore these lesions appear hyperenhanced against a minimally enhanced parenchymal background. Unfortunately, even with these optimized protocols there is still a large inter-patient variability regarding the degree of tumor en-

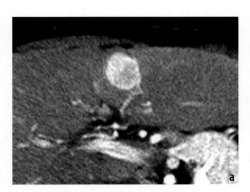

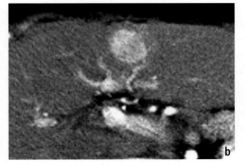

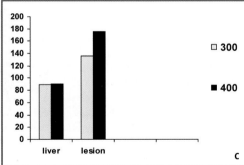

Fig. 6a-c. Higher-concentration of contrast medium (400 mg I/ml) (**a**) compared with a more conventional concentration (300 mg I/ml) (**b**) in the same patient leads to higher contrast enhancement of a nodule of hepatocellular carcinoma (HCC). Quantitative analysis (**c**) during the arterial phase shows that the mean hepatic enhancement was similar, while the difference in lesion density was about 40 Hounsfield units

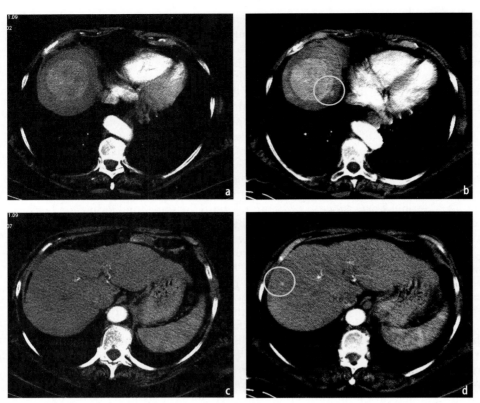

Fig. 7a-d. Comparison of 300 (**a, c**) and 400 (**b, d**) mg I/ml of contrast medium in the same patient. The enhancement of a large HCC is significantly higher with the more concentrated contrast medium (compare **b** and **a**). Moreover, two additional satellite nodules are demonstrated with the higher concentration (**b, d**)

hancement that can be obtained [18, 19]. We reported our experience in biphasic CT studies using a non-ionic contrast medium at an iodine concentration of 400 mg/ml [20]. A cross-over study design was chosen. Following local ethics committee approval, 22 consecutive patients with HCC underwent two complete sessions of biphasic spiral CT within a brief period, one scan with Iomeprol 300, the other with Iomeprol 400 as contrast agent. Comparison was made of patients given an equal iodine dose (45 g/patient) at a fixed rate of delivery (4 ml/s). Both lesion density, expressed as absolute value in Hounsfield units, and lesion-to-liver contrast (the difference of lesion density and parenchyma density in the same contrast phase) increased significantly more during the arterial phase at higher contrast medium concentration ($P=0.0016$ and $P=0.0005$, respectively, using ANOVA) (Fig. 6). In this limited number of patients, more lesions were detected with the more concentrated contrast medium during the arterial phase (42 vs. 37); however, this difference was not statistically significant (Fig. 7). During the portal venous phase no significant differences were observed. When the total iodine dose is fixed but a higher concentration and a lower volume of contrast medium is used, an earlier and higher arterial enhancement is obtained. Venous phase enhancement does not change because it is determined by the total given dose of iodine. As a result with this technique a greater diagnostic efficacy can be obtained without an increase in cost. A smaller volume of a more concentrated contrast medium seems to be the answer to a narrow time window for scanning [21].

A further approach to the optimization of spiral CT of the liver is the so-called saline push technique [22]. A substantial amount of contrast medium remains in the dead space of the injector tubing, peripheral veins, and central circulation. This amount of contrast does not contribute to image quality and is wasted. With the saline push technique a similar enhancement can be obtained with a lower volume or the enhancement can be improved if the amount is kept constant. Manufacturers have recently introduced a new line of power injectors specifically designed for use with a saline chaser.

Conclusions

In liver imaging, MDCT has many advantages over single-row CT. The high speed offers the possibility of thin-slice imaging during clearly defined contrast phases. With fast scanners, it is necessary to increase iodine administration rates but this rate is limited by the quality of the venous access. Therefore lower volumes at higher concentrations are likely to represent a good compromise.

References

1. el-Serag HB (2001) Epidemiology of hepatocellular carcinoma. Clin Liver Dis 5:87-107
2. Silverman PM, Kohan L, Ducic I et al (1998) Imaging of the liver with helical CT: a survey of scanning techniques. Am J Roentgenol 170:149-152
3. Hollett MD, Jeffrey RB Jr, Nino-Murcia M et al (1995) Dual-phase helical CT of the liver: value of arterial phase scans in the detection of small (< or = 1.5 cm) malignant hepatic neoplasms. AJR Am J Roentgenol 164:879-884
4. Baron RL, Oliver JH Jr, Dodd GD Jr et al (1996) Hepatocellular carcinoma: evaluation with biphasic, contrast-enhanced, helical CT. Radiology 199:505-511
5. Kopp AF, Heuschmid M, Claussen CD (2002) Multidetector helical CT of the liver for tumor detection and characterization. Eur Radiol 12:745-752
6. Kawata S, Murakami T, Kim et al (2002) Multidetector CT: diagnostic impact of slice thickness on detection of hypervascular hepatocellular carcinoma. AJR Am J Roentgenol 179:61-66
7. Foley WD, Mallisee TA (2000) Multiphase hepatic CT with a multidetector CT scanner. Am J Roentgenol 175:679-685
8. Murakami T, Kim T, Takaruma M et al (2001) Hypervascular hepatocellular carcinoma: detection with double arterial-phase multidetector-row-helical CT. Radiology 218:763-767
9. Ichikawa T, Kitamura T, Nakajima H et al (2002) Hypervascular hepatocellular carcinoma: can double arterial phase imaging with multidetector CT improve tumor depiction in the cirrhotic liver. AJR Am J Roentgenol 179:751-758
10. Laghi. A, Iannacone R, Rossi P et al (2003) Hepatocellular carcinoma: detection with a triple phase multidetector row helical CT in patients with chronic hepatitis. Radiology 226:543-549
11. Keogan MT, Seabourn JT, Paulson EK et al (1997) Contrast-enhanced CT of intrahepatic and hilar cholangiocarcinoma: delay time for optimal imaging. AJR Am J Roentgenol 169:1493-1499
12. Lim JH, Choi D, Kim SH et al (2002) Detection of hepatocellular carcinoma: value of adding delayed phase imaging to dual-phase helical CT. AJR Am J Roentgenol 179:961-968
13. Frederick MG, McElenay BL, Singer A et al (1996) Timing of parenchymal enhancement on dual-phase dynamic helical CT of the liver: how long does the hepatic phase predominate? AJR Am J Roentgenol 166:1305-1310
14. Brink JA (2003) Contrast optimization and scan timing for single and multidetector-row CT. J Comput Assist Tomogr 27 [Suppl 1]:3-8
15. Federle MP, Chang PJ, Confer S et al (1998) Frequency and effects of extravasation of ionic and non-ionic contrast media during rapid bolus injection. Radiology 206:637-640
16. Hänninen EL, Vogl TJ, Felfe R et al (2000) Detection of focal liver lesions at biphasic spiral CT: randomized, double-blind study of the effect of iodine concentration in contrast materials. Radiology 216:403-409
17. Awai K, Takada K, Onishi H et al (2002) Aortic and hepatic enhancement and tumor-to-liver contrast: analysis of the effect of different concentrations of contrast material at multidetector-row helical CT Radiology 224:757-763
18. Chambers T-P, Baron R-L, Lush R-M (1994) Hepatic CT enhancement. I. Alterations in the volume of contrast material within the same patients. Radiology 193:513-517
19. Chambers T-P, Baron R-L, Lush R-M (1994) Hepatic CT enhancement. II. Alterations in contrast material volume and rate of injection within the same patients. Radiology 193:518-522
20. Marchianò A, Spreafico C, Lanocita R et al (2004) Does iodine concentration affect the diagnostic efficacy of biphasic spiral CT in patients with hepatocellular carcinoma? Abdom Imaging (in press)
21. Silverman PM (2002) Optimizing contrast use in multislice CT. Appl Radiol [Suppl]:10-12
22. Dorio PJ, Lee FT, Hemseler M et al (2003) Using saline chaser to decrease contrast media in abdominal CT. AJR Am J Roentgenol 180:929-934

II.3

MDCT of the Pancreas

Jay P. Heiken

Introduction

With multidetector-row computed tomography (MDCT), images of the pancreas can be acquired with less than 1-mm collimation and viewed with reconstructed slice thickness ranging from 1 to 5 mm. Thus images are reconstructed from isotropic or nearly isotropic voxels, depending upon the specific acquisition parameters used. This technique enables very high-quality three-dimensional, multiplanar and curved planar reconstructions to be acquired. Consequently, large CT data sets can be viewed efficiently as volumes, rather than as individual transverse slices. The ability to view the image data as a volume also makes it easier to communicate the results efficiently to referring physicians, using a limited number of selected volume-rendered or multiplanar images. These images can be reconstructed to demonstrate the pancreatic duct, bile ducts, and peripancreatic vessels in a clinically relevant fashion.

MDCT Technique

Prior to imaging, patients drink approximately 1 l of fluid to opacify the stomach, duodenum, and jejunum. Water is preferred, rather than iodine or barium-based positive contrast materials, to avoid interference with volume-rendered reconstructions of the peripancreatic vessels. For the detection or staging of pancreatic adenocarcinoma, a volume of 150 ml of low-osmolar contrast material is administered at a rate of 5 ml/s [1, 2]. Images are acquired in two phases: a *pancreatic parenchymal phase* (beginning at 40–45 s from the start of contrast medium injection) and a *venous* or *hepatic parenchymal phase* (beginning 70 s from the start of contrast medium injection) [3, 4]. The pancreatic phase images are acquired with less than 1 mm collimation, whereas the venous phase im-

ages are acquired with 1.5-mm or 2.5-mm collimation, depending upon whether 4-detector or 16-detector CT is used (Tables 1 and 2). The images are reconstructed with 3-mm slice thickness at 2-mm intervals (1-mm slice thinkness at 1-mm intervals for 3D reconstructions). The data can be viewed on a workstation where three-dimensional volume-rendered, maximum intensity projection and multiplanar images can be viewed [5-9]. In addition, curved planar images can be constructed through key anatomical structures, such as the peripancreatic arteries and veins, the common bile duct, and the pancreatic duct [10, 11] (Figs. 1–5).

Adenocarcinoma of the Pancreas

MDCT is established as the primary initial imaging method for both the detection and staging of suspected pancreatic carcinoma. Most studies have found that CT is highly reliable when it demonstrates features indicating that a tumor is unresectable [12, 13]. The positive predictive value of a diagnosis of unresectability with single-detector helical CT (SDCT) has ranged from 92% to 100% [14, 18]. SDCT is less reliable, however, for predicting whether a tumor is resectable [negative predictive value (NPV) 76%–90%] [14–19]. In a recent study using eight-detector MDCT, the NPV and accuracy for vascular invasion were 100% and 99%, respectively [20]. The overall NPV in this study, however, was 87% due to undetected small hepatic and peritoneal metastases, which continue to be a limitation of CT, even MDCT.

Although criteria for unresectability vary among surgeons, imaging features that generally indicate unresectability include vascular invasion, lymph node metastases beyond those in the immediate vicinity of the pancreas, and distant metastases. Metastases most commonly involve the liver or peritoneum.

Table 1. 4-row MDCT

Pancreas: Dual Phase	
Indications	Evaluation of known or suspected pancreatic neoplasms Evaluation for complications of pancreatitis
Scan range	Pre-contrast: Standard abdomen Arterial: (craniocaudal) from third duodenum or inferior tip of liver, whichever is more caudal to the top of the pancreas. For suspected islet cell tumors, scan up to the diaphragm Venous: (craniocaudal) from iliac crest to diaphragm
mA selection	180-250 mA-adjust for patient size
Detector collimation	Pre-contrast: 2.5 mm Arterial: 1 mm Venous: 2.5 mm
Rotation time	0.5 s
Table speed (pitch)	Pre-contrast: 10–18 mm/rot (1-1.75) Arterial: 4–7 mm/rot (1-1.75) Venous: 13–18 mm/rot (1-1.75)
Slice thickness	Pre-contrast 5 mm Arterial: 3 mm and 1.25 mm (3-D) Venous: 3 mm
Reconstruction int.	3 mm for the 5-mm slices 1 mm for the 1.25-mm slices
IV contrast type	350–370 mgI/ml Volume: 150 ml Injection rate: 5 ml/s
Scan delay	Arterial: 40 s (for suspected islet cell tumors, this should be decreased to 30 s) Venous: 60 s (or ASAP)

Recent studies have demonstrated the usefulness of CT for evaluating vascular invasion by pancreatic carcinomas [20-24]. When a pancreatic tumor is not contiguous with a critical peripancreatic vessel such as the hepatic artery, superior mesenteric artery, superior mesenteric vein, or portal vein (i.e., when an intervening fat plane is present), vascular invasion is almost never present. When the tumor is contiguous with less than one-quarter of the vessel circumference, it is resectable in the majority of cases, but when the tumor is contiguous with one-quarter to one-half of the vessel circumference, it is unresectable in the majority of cases. It is in the group of patients in which the tumor con-

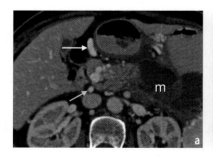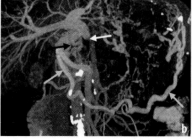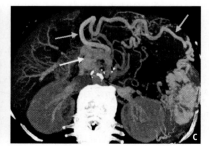

Fig. 1a-c. Unresectable pancreatic cancer. **a** The transaxial image demonstrates a large heterogeneous mass (*m*) involving the tail of the pancreas. The posterior superior pancreatoduodenal vein (*yellow arrow*) and the gastroepiploic vein (*white arrow*) are dilated, indicating invasion of the superior mesenteric vein and splenic vein, respectively. **b** A coronal maximum intensity projection image shows the dilated posterior superior pancreaticoduodenal vein (*black arrow*) and gastroepiploic vein (*yellow arrows*). The portal vein is occluded at its confluence with the superior mesenteric vein (*white arrow*). **c** A transaxial maximum intensity projection image also demonstrates the dilated posterior superior pancreaticoduodenal (*white arrow*) and gastroepiploic (*yellow arrows*) veins

Table 2. 16-row MDCT

Pancreas: Dual Phase	
Indications	Evaluation of known or suspected pancreatic neoplasms
	Evaluation for complications of pancreatitis
Scan range	Pre-contrast: standard abdomen
	Arterial: (craniocaudal) from diaphragm to bottom of liver
	Venous: (craniocaudal) from diaphragm to iliac crest
Effective mA	180
Detector collimation	Pre-contrast: 1.5 mm
	Arterial: 0.75 mm
	Venous: 1.5 mm
Rotation time	0.5 s
Table speed (pitch)	Pre-contrast: 24–30 mm/rot (1–1.25)
	Arterial: 12–15 mm/rot (1–1.25)
	Venous: 24–30 mm/rot (1–1.25)
Slice thickness	Pre-contrast 5 mm
	Arterial: 3 mm and 1 mm (3-D)
	Venous: 3 mm
Reconstruction int.	3 mm for the 5-mm slices
	0.8 mm for the 1-mm slices
IV contrast type	350–370 mgI/ml
	Volume: 150 ml
	Injection rate: 5 ml/s
Scan delay	Arterial: 45 s (for suspected islet cell tumors, this should be decreased to 35 s)
	Venous: 65 s (or ASAP)

tacts up to one-half of the vessel circumference that endoscopic ultrasonography may be of value in assessing vascular invasion. Otherwise, surgical exploration is needed to determine resectability. Tumors contacting more than one-half of the circumference of the vessel are nearly always unresectable. Another sign of unresectability of adenocarcinoma of the head of the pancreas is a teardrop shape of the superior mesenteric vein, which represents either direct tumor infiltration of the vein or peritumoral fibrosis adherent to the vessel [25].

Assessment of the peripancreatic veins can also provide information regarding the likelihood of vascular invasion by pancreatic carcinoma. In pa-

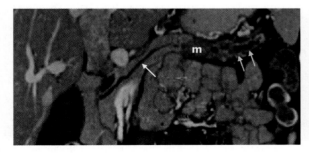

Fig. 2. Resectable pancreatic cancer. Curved planar reformation through the pancreatic duct demonstrates a mass (*m*) in the body of the pancreas. The tail of the pancreas is atrophic with a dilated pancreatic duct (*yellow arrows*). The pancreatic duct in the head and neck of the pancreas (*white arrow*) is normal

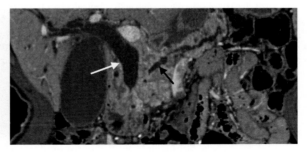

Fig. 3. Pancreatic adenocarcinoma. Curved planar reformatted image through the common bile duct (*white arrow*) and pancreatic duct (*black arrow*) shows obstruction of both ducts by an adenocarcinoma that diffusely infiltrates the pancreatic head

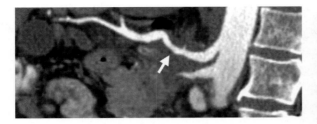

Fig. 4. Unresectable pancreatic carcinoma. Curved planar reformation through the hepatic artery (*arrow*) demonstrates that the vessel is encased by tumor

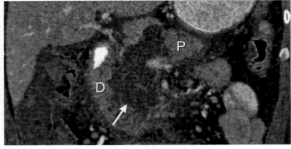

Fig. 5. Pancreatic necrosis in a patient with severe acute pancreatitis. Curved planar reformatted image through the pancreas shows necrosis of the pancreatic head and neck (*arrow; D* duodenum, *P* intact pancreatic parenchyma)

tients with pancreatic carcinoma, dilatation of the posterior superior pancreaticoduodenal vein or the gastrocolic trunk is a sign of portal or superior mesenteric vein invasion [26-29] (Fig. 1). However, a dilated gastrocolic trunk should not be used as an independent sign of surgical unresectability [24].

Pancreatitis

MDCT is the imaging method of choice for evaluating complications of acute and chronic pancreatitis. Three-dimensional, multiplanar, and curved planar reconstructions of the data are useful for demonstrating the extent of pancreatic necrosis (Fig. 5) and peripancreatic fluid collections, and for demonstrating intraductal pancreatic calculi. CT angiography is an excellent technique for delineating pseudoaneurysms of the peripancreatic vessels.

References

1. Tublin ME, Tessler FN, Cheng SL et al (1999) Effect of injection rate of contrast medium on pancreatic and hepatic helical CT. Radiology 210:97-101
2. Kim T, Murakami T, Takahashi S et al (1999) Pancreatic CT imaging: effects of different injection rates and doses of contrast material. Radiology 212:219-225
3. Lu DS, Vandantham S, Krasny RM et al (1996) Two-phase helical CT for pancreatic tumors: pancreatic versus hepatic phase enhancement of tumor, pancreas, and vascular structures. Radiology 199:697-701
4. Boland GW, O'Malley ME, Saez M et al (1999) Pancreatic-phase versus portal vein-phase helical CT of the pancreas: optimal temporal window for evaluation of pancreatic adenocarcinoma. AJR Am J Roentgenol 172:605-608
5. Raptopoulos V, Steer ML, Sheiman RG et al (1997) The use of helical CT and CT angiography to predict vascular involvement from pancreatic cancer: correlation with findings at surgery. AJR Am J Roentgenol 168:971-977
6. Baek SY, Sheafor DH, Keogan MT (2001) Two-dimensional multiplanar and three-dimensional volume-rendered vascular CT in pancreatic carcinoma: interobserver agreement and comparison with standard helical techniques. AJR Am J Roentgenol 176:1467-1473
7. Fishman EK, Horton KM, Urban BA (2000) Multidetector CT angiography in the evaluation of pancreatic carcinoma: preliminary observations. J Comput Assist Tomogr 24:849-853
8. Lepanto L, Arzoumanian Y, Glanfelice D et al (2002) Helical CT with CT angiography assessing periampullary neoplasms: identification of vascular invasion. Radiology 222:347-352
9. Nino-Murcia M, Tamm EP, Charnsangavej C et al (2003) Multidetector-row helical CT and advanced postprocessing techniques for the evaluation of pancreatic neoplasms. Abdom Imaging 28:366-377
10. Nino-Murcia M, Jeffrey RB, Beaulieu CF et al (2001) Multidetector CT of the pancreas and bile duct system: value of curved planar reformations. AJR Am J Roentgenol 176:689-693
11. Prokesch RW, Chow L, Beaulieu CF et al (2002) Local staging of pancreatic carcinoma with multidetector-row CT: use of curved planar reformation–initial experience. Radiology 224:764-768
12. Andrén-Sandberg A, Lindberg CG, Lundstedt C et al (1998) Computed tomography and laparoscopy in the assessment of the patient with pancreatic cancer. J Am Coll Surg 186:35-40
13. Freeny PC, Traverso LW, Ryan JA (1993) Diagnosis and staging of pancreatic adenocarcinoma with dynamic computed tomography. Am J Surg 165:600-605
14. Zeman RK, Cooper C, Zeiberg AS et al (1997) TNM staging of pancreatic carcinoma using helical CT. AJR Am J Roentgenol 169:459-464
15. Diehl SJ, Lehmann KJ, Sadick M et al (1998) Pancreatic cancer: value of dual-phase helical CT in assessing resectability. Radiology 206:373-378
16. Sheridan MB, Ward J, Guthrie JA et al (1999) Dynamic contrast-enhanced MR imaging and dual-phase helical CT in the preoperative assessment of suspected pancreatic cancer: a comparative study with receiver operating characteristic analysis. AJR Am J Roentgenol 173:583-590
17. Legmann P, Vignaux O, Dousset B et al (1998) Pancreatic tumors: comparison of dual-phase helical CT

and endoscopic sonography. AJR Am J Roentgenol 170:1315-1322

18. Coley SC, Strickland NH, Walker JD et al (1997) Spiral CT and the pre-operative assessment of pancreatic adenocarcinoma. Clin Radiol 52:24-30

19. Tabuchi T, Itoh K, Ohshio G et al (1999) Tumor staging of pancreatic adenocarcinoma using early and late-phase helical CT. AJR Am J Roentgenol 173:375-380

20. Vargas R, Nino-Murcia M. Trueblood W, Jeffrey RB (2004) MDCT in pancreatic adenocarcinoma: prediction of vascular invasion and resectability using a multiphasic technique with curved planar reformations. AJR Am J Roentgenol 182:419-425

21. Loyer EM, David CL, Dubrow RA et al (1996) Vascular involvement in pancreatic adenocarcinoma: reassessment by thin-section CT. Abdom Imaging 21:202-206

22. Lu DSK, Reber HA, Krasny RM et al (1997) Local staging of pancreatic cancer: criteria for unresectability of major vessels as revealed by pancreatic-phase, thin-section helical CT. AJR Am J Roentgenol 168:1439-1443

23. Furukawa H, Kosuge T, Mukai K et al (1998) Helical computed tomography in the diagnosis of portal vein invasion by pancreatic head carcinoma. Arch Surg 133:61-65

24. O'Malley ME, Boland GWL, Wood BJ et al (1999) Adenocarcinoma of the head of the pancreas: determination of surgical unresectability with thin-section pancreatic-phase helical CT. AJR Am J Roentgenol 173:1513-1518

25. Hough TJ, Raptopoulos V, Siewert B et al (1999) Teardrop superior mesenteric vein: CT sign for unresectable carcinoma of the pancreas. AJR Am J Roentgenol 173:1509-1512

26. Mori H, Miyake H, Aikawa H et al (1991) Dilated posterior superior pancreaticoduodenal vein: recognition with CT and clinical significance in patients with pancreaticobiliary carcinomas. Radiology 181:793-800

27. Mori H, McGrath FP, Malone DE et al (1992) The gastrocolic trunk and its tributaries: CT evaluation. Radiology 182:871-877

28. Hommeyer SC, Freeny PC, Crabo LG (1995) Carcinoma of the head of the pancreas: evaluation of the pancreaticoduodenal veins with dynamic CT–potential for improved accuracy in staging. Radiology 196:233-238

29. Yamada TJ, Mori H, Kiyosue H et al (2000) CT assessment of the inferior peripancreatic veins: clinical significance. AJR Am J Roentgenol 174:677-684

II.4

Abdominal Imaging: Use of High-Concentration Contrast Media

Renate M. Hammerstingl

Introduction

Computed tomography (CT) remains one of the main techniques for imaging of the hepatobiliary and pancreatic systems and for the diagnosis of focal liver lesions. It is still the most commonly used modality for the evaluation of focal liver lesions after initial sonography [1]. With the increasing use of CT, diagnostic accuracy has been dramatically enhanced resulting in detection rates of up to 95% for liver lesions larger than 1 cm. CT scanning of the pancreas is most commonly performed to image inflammatory pancreatic disease with its associated complications and to detect and characterize benign versus malignant pancreatic tumors [2].

Abdominal Imaging in MDCT

Since its clinical introduction in 1989, volumetric CT scanning has resulted in a revolution in diagnostic imaging. Spiral CT has improved over the last few years, with faster gantry rotation, more powerful X-ray tubes, and improved interpolation algorithms, but the greatest advance has been the introduction of multidetector-row CT (MDCT). Currently capable of acquiring 64 channels of helical data simultaneously, MDCT scanners have achieved the greatest incremental gain in scan speed and now enable rapid thin-section imaging of regional body anatomy [3]. Faster scanning creates the opportunity to image with increased speed, more reasonable breath-hold times, better image quality, and improved three-dimensional and multiplanar reconstructions (Table 1). MDCT is adapted to hepatic and pancreatic imaging to produce, under the appropriate clinical circumstances, a multipass multiplanar study obtained during defined circulatory phases so as to best outline the vasculature and to detect and characterize focal parenchymal lesions.

Table 1. Diagnostic advantages of MDCT of the hepatobiliary system

Shorter scan duration
Improved scanning of parenchymal organs:
• well-defined phase of enhancement, perfusion
Longer scan ranges
CT angiography:
• aorta, hepatic arteries, portal vein, mesenteric vessels
Thinner sections
Near-isotropic imaging:
• arbitrary imaging planes, MPR, 3D rendering

This results in improved lesion detection of abdominal tumors, relating to aspects of tumor size and to tissue-to-tumor contrast ratio. Enhancement characteristics of three-phasic scanning as well as thinner reconstructed sections allow an improved lesion characterization in MDCT imaging of the abdomen.

Phases of Scanning in MDCT

Detection of abdominal lesions is determined by conspicuity and is related to the degree of tumor-to-tissue contrast [4]. Since tumor characterization is mainly based on the lesion contrast, uptake during the different enhancement phases and scanning in sufficient phases are absolutely mandatory (Fig. 1).

With MDCT, the ability to scan through the entire upper abdomen in a few seconds allows acquisition of two separate imaging sets of the upper tract within the time generally regarded as the *dominant arterial phase*.

During the *early arterial phase* (~20 s after the start of injection), there is avid enhancement in the arterial vessels but relatively little enhance-

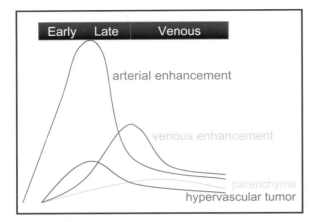

Fig. 1. Phases of scanning. Time-attenuation curves of different phases of hepatobiliary imaging. Arterial enhancement beginning at start of injection, venous enhancement at start of scanning

ment of the parenchyma or hypervascular lesions. Accurate CT angiography (CTA) with optimal vessel opacification can be performed for presurgical evaluation [5]. CTA provides detailed information on the vessel architecture and vascular characteristics of hypervascular lesions such as feeding arteries. Accurate delineation of the hepatic vascular anatomy allows segmental localization and assists in surgical and nonsurgical planning [6].

In the *late arterial phase* or portal venous *inflow phase*, which occurs approximately at 30-35 s after injection, solid neoplasms will be maximally enhanced, whereas the parenchyma will be only minimally enhanced due to predominantly portal venous supply. Therefore this phase is optimal for detection of hypervascular primary liver tumors and hypervascular metastatic infiltration. The *pancreatic parenchymal phase* begins at ~40-45 s after injection and provides the highest rates of enhancement of the pancreatic parenchyma.

The phase of portal venous dominance, the *hepatic venous phase* or *portal venous phase or hepatic parenchymal phase*, occurs ~60-70 s after the start of injection, with maximum enhancement of the hepatic parenchyma and high enhancement rates in the pancreatic parenchyma. During this phase, the detection of relatively hypovascular tumors is possible, such as colorectal metastases or adenocarcinoma of the pancreas, which may be unsuspected and in some cases poorly imaged during the other two phases.

Delayed-phase imaging (~8-10 min after injection) is used to provide additional information for the characterization of hypervascular lesions, such as hepatocellular or cholangiocellular carcinomas.

Multiphasic Contrast-Enhanced MDCT Imaging in the Liver

Detection

Optimal delineation of hypervascular liver lesions compared to surrounding liver parenchyma is established in the arterial phase of MDCT. Early arterial-phase imaging is distinguished from late arterial-phase scanning by *an increase of sensitivity for small hypervascular tumors*. Foley et al. [7] piloted the use of triple-phase contrast-enhanced hepatic imaging. They described three distinct circulatory phases: (a) the hepatic arterial phase; (b) the portal venous inflow phase or late arterial phase; and (c) the hepatic venous phase with a maximum of tumor-to-liver contrast, making this phase optimal for lesion detection. Using double arterial imaging, Murakami et al. [8], reported an increased detection rate of hepatocellular carcinoma (HCC), with a sensitivity of up to 86% and a positive predictive value of 92% (Fig. 2). Kadota and coworkers [9] described the use of both early and late arterial phases, with an increased detection rate of small HCC (87% sensitivity). Contrary to that, Ichikawa et al. [10] and Laghi et al. [11] found no significant improvement of double arterial-phase imaging compared to single late arterial-phase imaging. In a recently published study, Zhao et al. [12] highlighted these results, and in their series they observed no statistically significant difference between a double compared to a single arterial protocol in the late phase regarding the detection rate of HCC nodules.

Characterization

Enhancement patterns such as homogeneous fill-in, abnormal internal vessels, peripheral puddles, and a complete ring help to characterize lesions more precisely. According to Nino-Murcia and coworkers [13], abnormal internal vessels are associated with HCC, peripheral puddles with hemangioma, and a complete ring with metastasis with high sensitivity and specificity in arterial-phase CT studies (Fig. 3).

Triple-phase protocols in MDCT [14] depict the most common enhancement patterns of HCC, with hypervascularity in the arterial phase as well as a mosaic pattern on both arterial and portal venous images demonstrating wash-out.

Delayed-phase imaging is particularly important for differentiating HCC from cholangiocellular carcinoma (CCC) due to an increased tumor attenuation of CCC on delayed images compared to most HCCs [15].

According to Lim and coworkers [16], delayed-phase images were helpful in the characterization

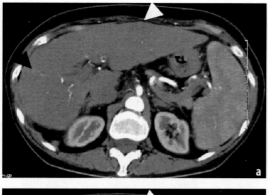

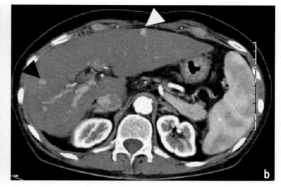

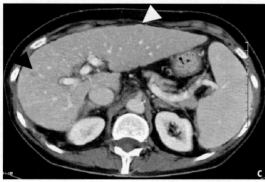

Fig. 2a-c. MDCT imaging of the liver: HCC and known hepatitis C. The early arterial phase (**a**) after i.v. injection of iomeprol 400 reveals a hypervascular HCC nodule (*black arrowhead*) in segment 8/7 of the right liver lobe. This nodule demonstrates increased density in the late arterial phase (**b**) and typical washout in the venous phase (**c**). A second HCC nodule (*white arrowhead*) is apparent on the late arterial (arterial inflow) phase image (**b**) but not on the early arterial (**a**) or venous (**c**) phase images. Additional high density regions suspicious for HCC are apparent only on the late arterial phase image

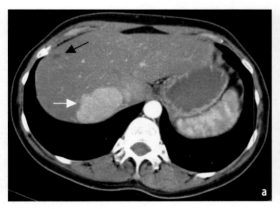

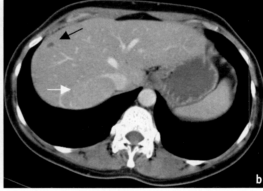

Fig. 3a, b. MDCT imaging of the liver: Simple cyst and FNH. In the arterial phase (**a**) a highly flushing tumor (*white arrow*) is depicted near the inferior vena cava. A second non-enhancing lesion (*black arrow*) is visualized in the right liver lobe. During the venous phase (**b**) the previously flushing lesion (*white arrow)* demonstrates near isodensity due to a significant decrease of attenuation which is typical of FNH. The second lesion (*black arrow*) shows no enhancement and is identified as a simple liver cyst

of HCC in 14% of their patient population, especially for hypovascular carcinomas (well differentiated or early HCC).

Multiphasic Contrast-Enhanced MDCT Imaging in the Pancreas

One main goal of pancreatic imaging is to identify the complications of acute pancreatitis after the disease has been diagnosed from laboratory test results [17]. There are three main complications of acute pancreatitis: pancreatic necrosis, pseudocyst formation, and pancreatic abscess [18]. Another aim of pancreatic imaging is tumor imaging (Fig. 4). The detection of tumorous tissue and visualization of organ as well as vessel infiltration, particularly in the superior mesenteric artery and vein, is important so as to determine whether a tumor is resectable or not [19]. For visualization of organ infiltration, a good contrast-to-noise ratio is mandatory (Fig. 5). To diagnose vessel infiltration, the optimal imaging phase must be timed.

According to Aschoff et al. [20], there is no need

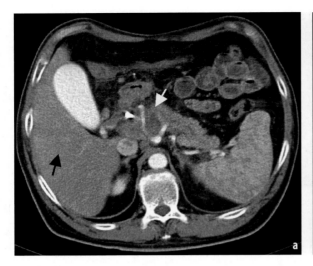
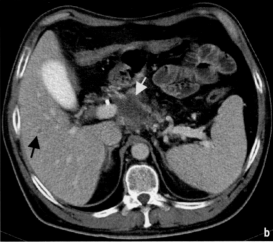

Fig. 4a, b. MDCT imaging of the pancreas: pancreatic carcinoma. A hypodense tumorous mass (*white arrow*) in the head of the pancreas with compression of the coelical trunk is appartent on both the arterial phase (**a**) and portal venous phase (**b**) images. Use of a high concentration contrast medium (Iomeprol 400 i.v.) permits the additional identification of a small hypodense liver metastasis (*black arrow*)

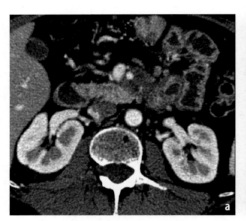
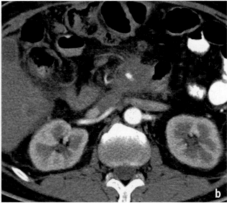

Fig. 5a, b. MDCT-Imaging of the pancreas: comparison of chronic pancreatitis and pancreatic carcinoma. Documentation of local chronic pancreatitis within the pancreatic corpus (**a**). There is no infiltration of the superior mesenteric artery. Delineation of encasement of the superior mensenteric artery in a pancreatic carcinoma (**b**)

to administer butylscopolamine to reduce bowel motion when using dual or multislice scanners, since there is no improvement in image quality.

A triple-phase protocol (unenhanced, arterial, and portal venous phases) is generally used for imaging of the pancreas. A more modern concept for pretherapeutic staging includes quadruple-phase scanning carrying out unenhanced, arterial, pancreatic parenchymal, and portal venous-phase imaging. The additional pancreatic parenchymal phase with a delay of ~35 s after contrast medium administration provides an optimal contrast-to-noise ratio of pancreatic tumors versus surrounding tissue. McNulty and coworkers [21] reported that the highest attenuation of normal pancreatic tissue occurred in the pancreatic parenchymal phase compared to the arterial and portal venous

phases, with a statistically significant difference compared to the arterial phase but not to the portal venous phase. The greatest enhancement in the celiac and superior mesenteric arteries occurs in the pancreatic parenchymal phase. For the superior mesenteric vein and the portal vein, contrast enhancement was highest in the portal venous phase. The tumors show up best in the pancreatic parenchymal phase and quite well in the portal venous phase. Imaging in the arterial phase is required for CTA to depict the vascular anatomy and diagnose disease [22]. According to Fishman and coworkers [23], a combination of CTA techniques and three-dimensional volume rendering allows one to create unique displays for evaluating pancreatic cancer and for accurate staging in these patients (Tables 2, 3).

Contrast Optimization

When imaging the abdomen, the depiction of soft tissue requires a certain amount of total iodine for appropriate scanning. The optimal amount of iodine should be around 35–45 g total volume of iodine. Taking a middle rate of 40 g of iodine per imaging into consideration, the following parameters should be used: For a lower-concentrated contrast agent (300 mg I/ml), an overall volume of 130 ml is necessary for adequate imaging quality; for 350 mg I/ml, 115 ml of contrast medium is needed; for 400 mg I/ml, 100 ml is used.

In addition, we should be aware of the fact that advances in CT technology also open the door to new approaches in the administration of iodinated contrast medium. Due to faster scanning in MDCT applications, the traditional concept for hepatic imag-

Table 2. Scanning protocol in MDCT of the hepatobiliary system (4-slice scanner)

Scan	Arterial phase	Portal venous phase
Collimation	4×1 mm	4×2.5 mm
Normalised pitch	1.5	1
Table feed/ gantry rotation	6 mm	10 mm
kV	120	120
Tube current (effective mAs)	150–180	150–180
Time of rotation (s)	0.5	0.5
Scan duration (s)	15	10
Scan delay:	CB (120 HU threshold)	
(post cm injection start)	~30 s	~60 s
Contrast concentration (mg l/ml)	370–400	
Contrast material (Volume in ml)	80	40
Injection rate (ml/s)	4	3
Saline flush (Volume in ml)	30–50	
MPR:		
Reconstruction (mm)	2	3
Increment (mm)	1	2
Scanner: Siemens Volume Zoom		

Table 3. Scanning protocol in MDCT of the hepatobiliary system (16-slice scanner)

Scan	Early arterial phase	Late arterial phase	Portal venous phase
Collimation	16×0.75 mm	16×1.5 mm	16×1.5 mm
Normalised pitch	1	1	1
Table feed/ gantry rotation	12 mm	24 mm	24 mm
kV	120	120	120 mm
Tube current (effective mAs)	150–180	150–180	50–180
Time of rotation (s)	0.5	0.5	0.5
Scan duration (s)	10	5	5
Scan delay:	CB (140 HU threshold)		
(post cm injection start)	~22 s	~40 s	~60 s
Contrast concentration (mg l/ml)	400		
Contrast material (Volume in ml)	60		30
Injection rate (ml/s)	4.5		2.5
Saline flush (Volume in ml)	30-50		
MPR:			
Reconstruction (mm)	1	2	2
Increment (mm)	0.5	1	1
Scanner: Siemens Sensation 16			

Table 4. Effects of contrast media in CT

Modulation of arterial enhancement
Injection rate of CM (iodine administration rate):
- doubling causes twice of enhancement
Injection duration:
- first pass and recirculation effects
- longer injections lead to continuously
increase of enhancement
Modulation of parenchymal enhancement
Determination of total CM volume (total iodine dose)
Independent of injection flow rate

ing, where the injection duration equals the speed of scanning, is no longer applicable. With this decreased period of scanning, the injection duration also has to be shortened and the iodine has to be delivered within seconds to ensure adequate vessel opacification as well as optimal parenchymal imaging (Table 4). One way of achieving this is to increase the injection speed, which is limited because of issues related to intravenous access. Another possibility to increase the iodine administration rate is to use a high concentration of lower-volume contrast agents [24-26].

Use of High-Concentration Contrast Media: Liver Imaging

According to Hanninen and colleagues [27], a decrease in iodine concentration significantly affects aortic and hepatic contrast enhancement and impairs the delineation of focal liver lesions during biphasic spiral CT. Hepatic time-attenuation curves and mean hepatic enhancement in the portal venous phase and aortic time-attenuation curves in both arterial and portal venous phases were statistically superior using Iopromide at a concentration of 370 mg Iodine/ml compared to 300 mg Iodine/ml. The same volumes were used in both groups, and therefore the total iodine amount was different.

Regarding the vascular system of the liver, a greater enhancement in the arterial vessels was documented with 300 mg I/ml versus 370 mg I/ml according to Spielmann and coworkers [28]. In this study, the total iodine dose was equal per group.

Concerning tumor imaging, Kim et al. [29] found a greater enhancement of HCC using higher-concentrated contrast media ($P<0.05$) in a protocol of 100 ml 370 mg I/ml and a flow rate of 4 ml/s compared to 100 ml of 300 mg I/ml and the same flow rate. A higher iodine delivery rate was administered to the patients using 1.48 compared to 1.2 g iodine per second.

Awai and coworkers [30] found that a higher concentration of contrast material is effective for a significantly higher tumor-to-liver contrast in arterial-phase imaging. An iodine concentration of 300 mg I/ml was compared with 370 mg I/ml. The same total load of iodine was used per patient and per body weight of patient. In the early arterial phase, a significant increase of aortic enhancement was documented ($P<0.01$) with a superior depiction of hepatic arteries and an increased tumor-to-liver contrast for the high-concentration contrast media.

In chronic liver disease, a higher iodine concentration (370 mg I/ml) was helpful for diagnostic imaging in the liver. Contrast enhancement of liver parenchyma was improved in the portal-phase and late-phase images with better overall image quality [31].

In a recent multicenter study presented at the 2003 annual meeting of the Radiological Society of North America, we reported our experience [32] from an abdominal study using a non-ionic contrast medium (Iomeprol) with an iodine concentration of 400 mg/ml compared to 300 and 350 mg/ml. In this double-blind, randomized, parallel-group comparison clinical study, 91 patients with the diagnosis of abdominal tumors were included. All patients underwent MDCT using a biphasic contrast-enhanced technique. Iomeprol was administered intravenously at three different concentrations via an automatic power injector. The overall iodine dose (36 g) was equal for each group. The injection rate for all three groups was 4 ml/s for arterial-phase imaging and 2 ml/s for portal venous-phase imaging. Higher contrast density values of normal liver tissue enhancement ($P<0.012$; Fig. 6) and pancreatic tissue ($P=0.471$; Fig. 7) were calculated in the arterial phase for high-concentration contrast medium. For hypervascular tumors, the maximum of absolute contrast to surrounding tissue was increased, providing a better delineation of the vascularity of lesions (Fig. 8).

Contrary to our data, there was no significant increase in hepatic enhancement for arterial-phase imaging according to Engeroff and coworkers [33], who used a concentration of 370 mg I/ml in their study.

Use of High-Concentration Contrast Media: Pancreatic Imaging

In a study by Kim and coworkers [34], the effects of the intravenous injection rate and dose of contrast material on pancreatic CT were evaluated. Both a higher dose and a faster injection rate increased the maximum pancreatic enhancement value. Accordingly, studies were performed using higher-concentrated contrast media for imaging of the pancreas.

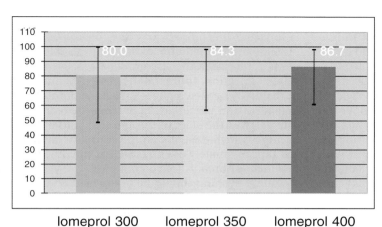

Fig. 6. Contrast density of normal liver tissue in the arterial phase. There was a statistically significant ($P=0.012$) increase of density of normal liver parenchyma in the arterial phase of imaging using the highest concentration of Iomeprol. The ANOVA test procedure was used for statistical analysis

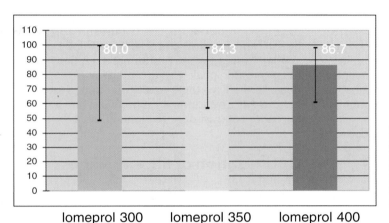

Fig. 7. Contrast density of pancreatic tissue in the arterial phase. There was an increase of density of pancreatic parenchyma in the arterial phase of imaging using the highest concentration of Iomeprol, although the results were not statistically significant ($P=0.471$). The Anova test procedure was used for statistical analysis

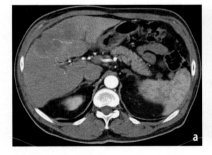
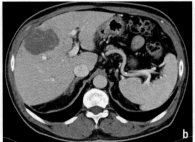
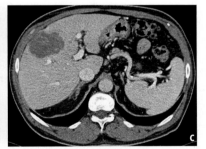

Fig. 8a-c. MDCT imaging of the liver: cholangiocellular carcinoma. Use of a high concentration contrast medium (Iomeprol 400 i.v.) permits clear depiction of both the feeding vessels and the hypervascularized rim of the tumor on the arterial phase image (**a**). The venous phase image (**b**) reveals a hypodense lesion with moderate enhancement in the periphery. The inner vascular perfusion is best visualized using thinner slices (**c**)

Merkle and coworkers [35] documented in their series a statistically significant difference in contrast enhancement using high-concentration contrast medium (Iomeprol 400 mg I/ml). In arterial-phase imaging, higher attenuation values were calculated for the superior mesenteric artery and celiac trunk ($P<0.01$) as well as for the pancreas, right and left kidney, and spleen ($P<0.01$) in addition to the portal vein and liver ($P>0.01$). In venous-phase scanning, a significant difference in pancreatic enhancement was depicted. There was an improvement in the contribution of high-concentration contrast media toward diagnostic value ($P=0.02$), technical quality ($P=0.02$), and evaluability of vessels in arterial-phase imaging.

Fenchel et al. [36] evaluated the influence of two different iodine concentrations of the nonionic contrast agent Iomeprol, in iodine concentrations of 300 mg/ml and 400 mg/ml, on contrast enhancement of the pancreas. The overall iodine amount was equal per group. Iomeprol 400 led to significantly greater enhancement in the aorta, superior mesenteric artery, celiac trunk, pancreas, pancreatic carcinomas, kidneys, spleen, and wall of the small intestine than did Iomeprol 300. Portal venous-phase enhancement was significantly greater in the pancreas, pancreatic carcinomas, wall of the small intestine, and portal vein with Iomeprol 400. Two independent readers considered Iomeprol 400 superior to Iomeprol 300 concerning the contribution of the contrast agent to the diagnostic value in pancreatic imaging.

The group of Shinagawa et al. [37] evaluated the maximum of enhancement in the pancreas using CT in patients with abdominal disease. The peak enhancement value of the pancreas was significantly greater with a concentration of 370 mg I/ml, a dose of 1.5 ml/kg, and a flow rate of 5 ml/s. Higher attenuation values were documented using a higher injection rate and higher iodine concentration due to the fact that pancreatic CT enhancement is more dependent on the dose of iodine per second than on the total iodine.

In conclusion, a fast injection rate and use of high-concentrated contrast medium provides a greater enhancement of the pancreas and allows better diagnostic imaging (Fig. 9).

Optimization of Injection Technique

Determination of the circulation time is of great importance. In patients with low cardiac output, fixed scan delays are not appropriate for optimal phase scanning and characterization of focal liver lesions. A change in cardiac output affects aortic and hepatic enhancement. A decrease in cardiac output will delay aortic and hepatic peak enhancement.

A test bolus can be used to calculate the circulation time. It is more convenient to use a care bolus technique either with automatic thresholds (region of interest in the abdominal aorta; automatic start of injection, approximately 140 HU) (Table 5) or manually by viewing the contrast in the abdominal aorta and personally activating the scanning. The delay of the start of the spiral should be kept in mind, which depends on the scanner system itself (approximately 6-7 s), as well as the time to be included for breath-hold commands.

Saline flushing should be performed after contrast medium injection. A saline bolus washes out the residual contrast in the venous system, effectively leading to an increase of hepatic contrast enhancement for the same amount of contrast medium. A new line of power injectors has recently been introduced, designed specifically to permit the double injection of both contrast medium and saline flush. Zandrino and coworkers [38] documented similar timing for maximum aortic enhancement but a greater peak enhancement using a saline flush. In the liver there was earlier and greater enhancement. The administration of a saline bolus allowed for contrast dose reduction (Table 6).

Optimization of Slice Thickness

Thin sections can now be used on a routine basis in a single-breath-hold technique. Weg and coworkers [39] reported an increase in detection rates of 46% using thin sections for diagnostic imaging. However, Haider et al. [40] and Kawata et al. [41] found no improvement in the detection of focal liver lesions for slices thinner than 5 mm due to the increased noise. Kopka et al. [42] documented an overall detection rate of 96% and a characterization of focal liver lesions with a specificity of 87% using sections of 2- to 4-mm slice thickness

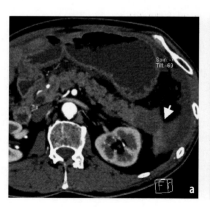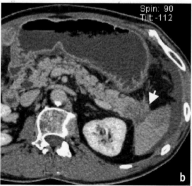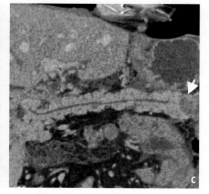

Fig. 9. MDCT-Imaging of the pancreas: pancreatic carcinoma. Distal parts of the pancreatic tail demonstrate on infiltrating adenocarcinoma (*white arrow*) in the arterial phase (**a**) and venous phase (**b**) of imaging (Iomeprol 400). Curved reconstruction of the pancreatic duct system documents very well the occlusion of the ductal parts due to tumour infiltration in venous imaging (**c**)

Table 5. Timing of scanning. Optimization of injection technique

Determination of circulation time
Test bolus: - precontrast scanning (20 ml of contrast media)   - calculation of circulation time
Care bolus technique:
Manual: - viewing of contrast in abdominal aorta
Automatic: - region of interest: abdominal aorta   - positioning: level of the coeliac trunc   - treshold: approx. 140 HU
Delay of scanner to start imaging: approx 6–7 s
Saline flushing post contrast media injection: 30-50 ml

Table 6. Spiral CT: abdominal imaging. Comparison of single slice and multislice CT regarding contrast material administration

Scanner	1-SCT	4-SCT	16-SCT
Contrast material volume (ml)	150	120	90–120
Contrast material concentration (mg l/ml)	300–350	350–400	370–400
Saline volume (ml)	30–50	30–50	30–50
Injection rate (ml/s) arterial/venous	3–4 ml	3–4 ml 2 ml	3–5 ml 2 ml

due to better visualization of enhancement of the inner structures, boundary, and rim. The higher noise is one drawback in the use of thinner sections, which has to be overcome (Fig. 10). Normalization of noise is mandatory for further study.

3D Imaging

Routine use of thin collimation and near-isotropic image acquisition allows the reconstruction of high-resolution multiplanar slices with the advantage of precise delineation of focal liver lesions. The capabilities of workstations make feasible the practical use of advanced post-processing techniques to create high-quality volumetric imaging: maximum intensity projections, volume rendering, curved planar reformations, and multiplanar reconstructions [43].

Kamel et al. [44] reported on the additional value of advanced image processing of multiplanar volume rendering and maximum intensity projec-

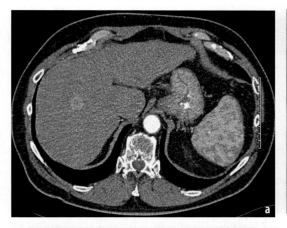
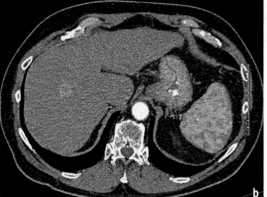
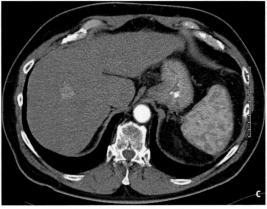

Fig. 10. MDCT-Imaging of the liver: hepatocellular carcinoma. Reduction of noise by using reduced effective slice thickness from 1 mm (**a**) to 3 mm (**b**) to 5 mm (**c**)

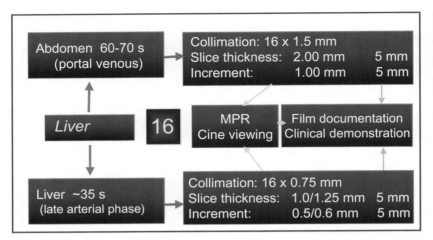

Fig. 11. MDCT-Imaging in the liver. Standard scanning protocol using 16-slice Scanner (Sensation 16, Siemens). Documentation of effective slice thickness for clinical demonstration, film documentation, cine viewing, and MPR reconstructions

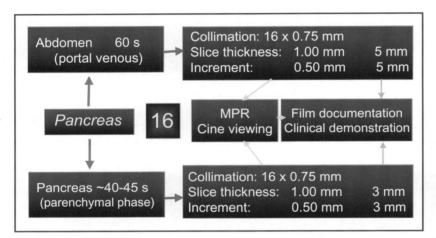

Fig. 12. MDCT-Imaging in the pancreas. Standard scanning protocol using a 16-slice Scanner (Sensation 16, Siemens). Documentation of effective slice thickness for clinical demonstration, film documentation, cine viewing, and MPR reconstructions

tion for hepatic imaging. Early detection of neovascularity and tumor stain as well as tumor burden is assessed better with these images than with routine axial images. Lesion characterization was also potentially improved with an accurate delineation of the hepatic vascular anatomy allowing segmental localization and providing assistance in surgical and nonsurgical planning (Fig. 11).

Prokesch and coworkers [45] found that the additional information of curved reformations greatly improved the diagnosis of pancreatic disease, but these reconstruction should not substitute transverse imaging (Fig. 12).

Conclusions

Over the last decade, major advances have occurred in CT. The speed and flexibility of MDCT have led to improvements in abdominal imaging, particularly related to the detection and characterization of abdominal masses.

MDCT scanning times may vary substantially in daily clinical routine use depending on the scanner type, and therefore acquisition parameters have to be modified. To ensure adequate vessel opacification as well as optimal detection and classification of hepatobiliary disease with fast MDCT acquisitions, the iodine administration rate needs to be increased. This can be achieved either by an increase of injection flow rate or - more conveniently - by using a higher iodine concentration of the contrast medium. These agents produce better enhancement of vascular structures and improved overall display of soft-issue tumors. This results in improved lesion detection relating to aspects of tumor size and to the surrounding tissue-to-tumor contrast ratio. Accurate scanning in optimal phases as well as thinner slices allow better characterization of hepatobiliary lesions. High-concentration contrast media show advantages in the demarcation and delineation of lesions compared to lower iodine-concentrated contrast agents, especially for the diagnosis of hypervascularized lesions.

References

1. Itoh S, Ikeda M, Achiwa M et al (2003) Multiphase contrast-enhanced CT of the liver with a multislice CT scanner. Eur Radiol 13:1085-1094
2. Foley WD, Kerimoglu U (2004) Abdominal MDCT: liver, pancreas, and biliary tract (review). Semin Ultrasound CT MR25:122-144
3. Prokop M (2003) General principles of MDCT. EUR J Radiol 45[Suppl 1]:4-10
4. Kopp AF, Heuschmid M, Claussen CD (2002) Multidetector helical CT of the liver for tumor detection and characterization. Eur Radiol 12:745-753
5. Sahani D, Saini S, Pena C et al (2002) Using multidetector CT for preoperative vascular evaluation of liver neoplasms: technique and results. AJR Am J Roentgenol 179:53-59
6. Rubin GD (2003) MDCT imaging of the aorta and peripheral vessels (review). Eur J Radiol [Suppl 1]:S42-S49
7. Foley WD, Mallisee TA, Hohenwalter MD et al (2000) Multiphase hepatic CT with a multirow detector CT scanner. AJR Am J Roentgenol 175:679-685
8. Murakami T, Kim T, Takamura M et al (2001) Hypervascular hepatocellular carcinoma: detection with double arterial phase multi-detector row helical CT. Radiology 218:763-767
9. Kadota M, Yamashita Y, Nakayama Y et al (1999) Valuation of small hepatocellular carcinoma with multidetector-row helical CT of the liver: the value of dual phase arterial scanning. Radiology (Book of abstracts, RSNA, p 124)
10. Ichikawa T, Kitamura T, Nakajima H et al (2002) Hypervascular hepato-cellular carcinoma: can double arterial phase imaging with multidetector CT improve tumor depiction in the cirrhotic liver? AJR Am J Roentgenol 179:751–758
11. Laghi A, Iannaccone R, Rossi P et al (2003) Hepatocellular carcinoma: detection with triple-phase multi-detector row helical CT in patients in chronic hepatitis. Radiology 226:543–549
12. Zhao H, Yao JL, Han MJ et al (2004) Multiphase hepatic scans with multirow-detector helical CT in detection of hypervascular hepatocellular carcinoma. Hepatobiliary Pancreat Dis Int 3:204-208
13. Nino-Murcia M, Olcott EW, Jeffrey RB Jr et al (2000) Focal liver lesions: pattern-based classification scheme for enhancement at arterial phase CT. Radiology 215:746-751
14. Lee KH, O`Malley ME, Haider MA et al (2004) Triple-phase MDCT of hepatocellular carcinoma. AJR Am J Roentgenol 182:643-649
15. Loyer EM, Chin H, DuBrow RA et al (1999) Hepatocellular carcinoma and intrahepatic peripheral cholangiocarcinoma: enhancement patterns with quadruple phase helical CT - a comparative study. Radiology 212:866-875
16. Lim JH, Choi D, Kim SH et al (2002) Detection of hepatocellular carcinoma: value of adding delayed phase imaging to dual-phase helical CT. AJR Am J Roentgenol 179:67-73
17. Balthazar EF (2002) Staging of acute pancreatitis. Radiol Clin N Am 40:1199-1209
18. Kim T, Murakami T, Takamura M et al (2001) Pancreatic mass due to chronic pancreatitis: correlation of CT and MR imaging features with pathologic findings. AJR Am J Roentgenol 177:367-371s
19. Horton KM, Fishman EK (2002) Adenocarcinoma of the pancreas. Radiol Clin N Am 40:1263-1272
20. Aschoff AJ, Gorich J, Sokiranski R (1999) Pancreas: does hyoscyamine butylbromide increase diagnostic value of helical CT? Radiology 210:861-864
21. McNulty NJ, Francis IR, Platt JF et al (2001) Multidetector row helical CT of the pancreas: effect of contrast-enhanced multiphasic imaging on enhancement of the pancreas, peripancreatic vasculature, and pancreatic adenocarcinoma. Radiology 220:97-102
22. Horton KM, Fishman EK (2002) Multidetector CT angiography of pancreatic carcinoma. AJR Am J Roentgenol 178:827-838
23. Fishman EK, Horton KM, Urban BA (2000) Multidetector CT angiography in the evaluation of pancreatic carcinoma: preliminary observations. J Comput Assist Tomogr 24:849-853
24. Fleischmann D (2003) Use of high-concentration contrast media in multiple-detector-row CT: principles and rationale. Eur Radiol 13[Suppl 5]:14-20
25. Brink JA (2003) Contrast optimization and scan timing for single and multidetector-row computed tomography. J Comput Assist Tomogr 27[Suppl 1]:S3-8
26. Bae KT, Heiken JP, Brink JA (1998) Aortic and hepatic peak enhancement at CT: effect of contrast medium injection rate - pharmacokinetic analysis and experimental porcine model. Radiology 206:455-464
27. Hanninen EL, Vogl TJ, Felfe R (2000) Detection of focal liver lesions at biphasic spiral CT: randomized double-blind study of the effect of iodine concentration in contrast materials. Radiology 216:403-409
28. Spielmann AL (2003) Liver imaging with MDCT and high concentration contrast media. Eur J Radiol 45 [Suppl 1]:50-52
29. Kim KA, Park CM, Lee W et al (2001) Small hepatocellular carcinoma: three-phase helical CT findings and pathologic correlation. Radiology 221:490 (Abstract book, RSNA)
30. Awai K, Takada K, Onishi H et al (2002) Aortic and hepatic enhancement and tumor-to-liver contrast: analysis of the effect of different concentrations of contrast material at multidetector-row helical CT. Radiology 224:757-763
31. Furuta A, Ito K, Fujita T et al (2004) Hepatic enhancement in multiphasic contrast-enhanced MDCT: comparison of high- and low-iodine concentration contrast medium in same patients with chronic liver disease. AJR Am J Roentgenol 183:157-162
32. Hammerstingl RM, Valette PJ, Regent DM et al (2003) Multidetector CT in abdominal imaging: optimization of iodine concentration for the diagnosis of abdominal tumors. Radiology (Book of abstracts, RSNA, p 413)
33. Engeroff B, Kopka L, Harz C et al (2001) Impact of different iodine concentrations on abdominal enhancement in biphasic multislice helical CT (MSCT). Rofo Fortschr Geb Rontgenstr Neuen Bildgeb Verfahr 173:938-941
34. Kim T, Murakami T, Takahashi S et al (1999) Pancreatic CT imaging: effects of different injection rates and doses of contrast material. Radiology 212:219-225
35. Merkle EM, Boll DT, Fenchel S (2003) Helical computed tomography of the pancreas: potential impact

of higher concentrated contrast agents and multidetector technology. JCAT 27[Suppl 1]:17-22

36. Fenchel S, Fleiter TR, Aschoff AJ et al (2004) Effect of iodine concentration of contrast media on contrast enhancement in multislice CT of the pancreas. Br J Radiol 77:821-830

37. Shinagawa M, Uchida M, Ishibashi M et al (2003) Assessment of pancreatic CT enhancement using a high concentration of contrast material. Radiat Med 21:74-79

38. Zandrino F, Musante F, Feretti MM et al (2001) Optimal contrast agent administration protocol for hepatic and aortic multidetector row computer tomography (MDCT): experience with two contrast agents at different injection rates. Radiology (Book of abstracts, RSNA, p 388)

39. Weg N, Scheer MR, Gabor MP (1998) Liver lesions: improved detection with dual-detector-array CT and routine 2.5 mm thin collimation. Radiology 209(2):417-426

40. Haider MA, Amitai MM, Rappaport DC, O'Malley ME, Hanbidge AE (2002) Multi-detector row helical CT in preoperative assessment of small (< or = 1.5 cm) liver metastases: is thinner collimation better? Radiology 225:137-142

41. Kawata S, Murakami T, Kim T et al (2002) Multidetector CT: diagnostic impact of slice thickness on detection of hypervascular hepatocellular carcinoma. AJR Am J Roentgenol 179:61-66

42. Kopka L, Rodenwaldt J, Hamm B (2000) Biphasic multi-slice helical CT of the liver: intra-individual comparison of different slice thicknesses for the detection and characterization of focal liver lesions. Radiology (Book of abstracts, RSNA, p 367)

43. Takeshita K, Furui S, Takada K (2002) Multidetector row helical CT of the pancreas: value of three-dimensional images, two-dimensional reformations and contrast-enhanced multiphasic imaging. J Hepatobiliary Pancreat Surg 9:576-582

44. Kamel IR, Lawler LP, Fishman EK (2004) Comprehensive analysis of hypervascular liver lesions using 16-MDCT and advanced image processing. AJR Am J Roentgenol 183:443-452

45. Prokesch RW, Chow LC, Beaulieu CF et al (2002) Local staging of pancreatic carcinoma with multidetector row CT: use of curved planar reformations initial experience. Radiology 225:759-765

SECTION III

Cardiac and Vascular Imaging

III

Introduction

Steven Dymarkowski and Johan de Mey

In the past few years multidetector-row computed tomography (MDCT) systems with simultaneous acquisition of multiple thin collimated slices and half-second scanner rotation have become widely available. CT scanners with 4 or more, and even up to 64 detector rows are widely used in clinical practice. MDCT represents a significant advance over single-slice detector CT since it allows rapid assessment of large areas of the body. The increased number of simultaneously acquired slices and sub-millimeter collimation allows true isotropic scanning with higher spatial, contrast, and temporal resolution. Experimental prototypes of flat-panel CT scans can already depict the entire heart in one simple gantry rotation with a pitch factor of 0.2 mm. MDCT has changed CT from a cross-sectional to a three-dimensional tool. It has become the new CT standard and its technical abilities are rapidly expanding the spectrum of application with clinically relevant examinations that were previously not possible with conventional scanning.

Due to the increased number of slices in 16-slice and 64-slice CT systems, dose utilization is improved compared with 4-slice CT scanners, and sub-millimeter collimation need no longer be restricted to special applications. Isotropic voxel data enable us to obtain sagittal and coronal images with a spatial resolution that is identical to axial images. Excellent volume data, which are acquired by MDCT, generate serviceable three-dimensional images using various reconstruction methods, such as multiplanar reconstruction (MPR), maximum intensity projection (MIP), minimum intensity projection, surface rendering, volume rendering, and virtual endoscopy.

The increased scan speed of MDCT systems can be used to cover an entire cardiac volume in one single, short breath-hold period, producing an isotropic data set free of cardiac motion if combined with retrospective cardiac triggering. Although the usefulness of MDCT for visualization of coronary arteries has been reported with 4- or 8-row CT systems, initial results from studies with 16-slice MDCT systems suggest that this technology not only offers the possibility of accurately visualizing coronary stenoses non-invasively but also of studying plaque morphology. The clinical performance of coronary CT angiography has certainly been substantially improved, allowing visualization of smaller coronary segments, coronary calcifications, and coronary stents. In the future, MDCT will be used to screen patients prior to cardiac catherization and to eliminate many unwarranted invasive procedures.

The technical developments of MDCT have also dramatically changed the application of CTA outside of the heart. The possibility of acquiring a large isotropic scanning range with thin slices without any loss in spatial resolution has revolutionized the assessment of abdominal vascular pathologies. With 4-detector row CT scanners the scan volume had to be focused on one specific abdominal vessel territory; 16-detector row technology now allows full abdominal coverage from the diaphragm to the groin with full spatial resolution. Therefore, comprehensive CTA of the abdomen can be performed without the necessity of focusing on any vascular territory. This technique enables the evaluation of the whole arterial visceral vasculature (e.g., hepatic vessels, mesenteric vessels, renal arteries) and the aortic–iliac axis in a single data acquisition. It allows investigation of the entire aorta and branch vessels in the evaluation of aneurysm, the thoracic aorta and the coronary arteries in cases of dissection, or the vascular and non-vascular chest in those with acute chest pain. MDCT has become critical for the pre-procedure planning and follow-up of several endovascular procedures, including endovascular aneurysm repair, lower extremity revascularization, and renal artery revascularization. The high sensitivity and negative predictive values reported in the literature are particularly promising for the use of MDCT in the evaluation of abdominal artery stenosis.

Limitations of single-splice spiral CT in the accurate diagnosis of isolated peripheral pulmonary embolism (PE) have so far prevented the acceptance of spiral CT as the new standard of reference for imaging PE. Concerns about the accuracy of spiral CT for the detection of PE may be overcome by the use of MDCT. The high spatial resolution allows evaluation of pulmonary vessels down to sixth-order branches and significantly increases the detection rate of segmental and subsegmental pulmonary emboli. Shorter breath-hold times also benefit patients with underlying lung disease and reduce the percentage of non-diagnostic CT scans. The true accuracy of multidetector-row spiral CT for the detection of small peripheral emboli in patients with suspected PE remains, however, difficult to determine, since as a direct result of high-resolution imaging capabilities, small peripheral clots that may have gone unnoticed in the past are now frequently seen, often in patients with minor symptoms. MDCT has nevertheless become an attractive means for a safe, highly accurate, cost-effective diagnosis of acute PE and may provide alternative diagnoses and explanations for symptoms in the absence of PE. It is emerging as a preferred modality for imaging patients with suspected acute PE and now challenges catheter pulmonary angiography, once the standard of reference, for the accurate detection of PE.

With increasingly faster acquisition speeds, contrast medium delivery is becoming increasingly difficult. The volume, concentration, and rate of injection, all affect the degree of enhancement that is achieved with an injection of contrast material. While the arterial enhancement is governed by injection speed and iodine concentration, the magnitude of enhancement in parenchymal organs is related primarily to the amount of iodine that accumulates in the extravascular space, independent of the speed of the CT scanner. Since the high speed of the MDCT scanner allows the recording of image data over a short time period, modifications of total iodine dose are best achieved by increasing iodine contrast concentration, rather than increasing the total volume of medium injected. Particular attention to methods of automated saline flushing and dual injection speed protocols can further refine the quality of MDCT examinations.

Many clinicians and researchers working in the cardiovascular field are still unfamiliar with the radiation doses that are received during MDCT examinations. Radiation doses received from specific MDCT protocols need to be evaluated. A second consideration is what to do with the detected pathology; are those small solitary vessel occlusions in pulmonary or other regions really relevant? More studies are necessary. We as radiologists must be careful to make a diagnosis with the least radiation possible and not to focus on beautiful images alone.

Although MDCT offers a decreased scan time, the reporting time is the main problem in the new radiological department. Huge amounts of data necessitate intelligent computer-aided viewing, reconstruction, quantification, and even real diagnostic support. MPR and MIP are still the standard tools but are insufficient for real vascular imaging. MDCT and a workstation with volume-rendering techniques can provide image quality that is superior to conventional angiography. Dedicated vessel-viewing tools can help to reduce reporting time and can aid in lesion quantification. It can be cost effective and it can improve diagnostic quality to invest in these workstations as well as three-dimensional vessel-viewing software and quantification tools.

MDCT continues to make amazing technical advancements in cardiovascular and body imaging and is currently experiencing a steadily increasing popularity based on the increase in diagnostic capabilities it has presented.

Suggested Reading

Knollmann F, Pfoh A (2003) Coronary artery imaging with flat-panel computed tomography. Circulation 107:1209

Juergens KU, Grude M, Maintz D et al (2004) Multi-detector row CT of left ventricular function with dedicated analysis software versus MR imaging: initial experience. Radiology 230:403-410

Wu AS, Pezzullo JA, Cronan JJ et al (2004) CT pulmonary angiography: quantification of pulmonary embolus as a predictor of patient outcome–initial experience. Radiology 230:831-835

Catalano C, Fraioli F, Laghi A et al (2004) Infrarenal aortic and lower-extremity arterial disease: diagnostic performance of multi-detector row CT angiography. Radiology 231:555-563

Schoepf UJ, Goldhaber SZ, Costello P (2004) Spiral computed tomography for acute pulmonary embolism. Circulation 109:2160-2167

III.1

Essentials of Contrast Medium Delivery for CT Angiography

Dominik Fleischmann

Introduction

Optimal intravenous CM injection remains one of the most crucial but difficult aspects of MDCT. Since the introduction of 8- and 16-channel MDCT systems, it has become evident that faster acquisitions can be used to advantage, but that they are less forgiving at the same time, and one may completely miss the bolus (e.g., in CTA) if CM injections are not adapted to the new scanner capabilities. This problem will become even more relevant with recently introduced 32-, 40-, and 64-channel scanners.

The purpose of this chapter is to review the physiological and pharmacokinetic principles governing vascular enhancement after intravenous CM administration. As opposed to the rapid evolution of scanner technology, these principles have not changed in the past, and most likely will not do so in the future. The effects of user-selectable injection parameters (CM injection rate, injection duration, and volume), CM concentration, injection devices (power injectors, saline flushing), and tools for scan timing (bolus triggering) will all be discussed, in order to provide the reader with the necessary tools for optimizing injection strategies for current and future cardiovascular applications of MDCT.

Pharmacokinetic and Physiological Principles

From a pharmacokinetic point of view, all angiographic X-ray CM represent extracellular fluid markers. After intravenous administration these agents are rapidly distributed between the vascular and interstitial compartments of the extracellular space [1]. For the time frame relevant to cardiovascular MDCT and CTA, it is this particularly complex early distribution/redistribution phase – or early CM dynamics – that determines vascular enhancement.

At this point it is essential to bear in mind the fundamental difference between injections aimed at vascular enhancement (CTA) and those aimed at parenchymal (e.g., hepatic) enhancement: Whereas early vascular enhancement is controlled by the relationship between iodine administration per unit of time (mg I/s) and blood flow per unit of time [i.e., cardiac output (l/min)], parenchymal enhancement is governed by the relationship between total iodine dose (mg I) and the total volume of distribution [i.e., body weight (kg)].

Recently, mathematical models have been developed to describe early vascular and parenchymal CM dynamics [2-4]. Such models are particularly useful to predict and illustrate the effects of different injection strategies, thus allowing for a more rational design of empiric, routinely applicable injection techniques.

Early Arterial CM Dynamics

Whereas time attenuation responses to intravenously injected CM vary widely between vascular territories and across individuals, some basic principles apply to all arterial (pulmonary and systemic) vessels. A first step towards a more intuitive understanding of the effects of vascular enhancement is to think in terms of *CM injection rate* and *injection duration*, rather than injection rate and CM volume.

Figure 1 illustrates the early arterial CM dynamics as observed in the abdominal aorta [5]. When a 16-ml test bolus of CM is injected intravenously, it causes an arterial enhancement response in the aorta (Fig. 1a, b). The time interval needed for the CM to arrive in the arterial territory of interest is referred to as the CM transit time (t_{CMT}). The first peak in the enhancement response is referred to as the "*first pass*" effect. The tail of the enhancement curve is due to bolus broadening and in part to recirculation. For a given individual and vascular territory, this enhancement response is proportional to the iodine injection rate. Hence, doubling the injection rate leads to twice the enhancement and requires twice the CM volume (Fig. 1c, d).

After the CM is distributed throughout the intravascular and interstitial fluid compartments of the body, a certain proportion of CM reenters the right heart ("*recirculation*"). This occurs fairly rapidly and therefore one will not only observe the *first pass* of contrast material but also its *recirculation* effect within the time frame of a CTA acquisition. Recirculation and bolus broadening have a profound effect on vascular enhancement when prolonged injections – such as in CT – are used. Figure 1e, f shows that a larger (128 ml), prolonged (32 s) bolus of CM can be viewed as the sum of eight subsequent injections of small "test boluses" of 16 ml each. Each of these eight "test boluses" has its own effect (first pass and recirculation) on arterial enhancement. Thus, the cumulative enhancement response to the entire 128-ml injection equals the sum (time integral) of each enhancement response to each of the eight test boluses [5]. The recirculation effects of the earlier test boluses overlap (and thus are additive) with the first pass effects of later test boluses. This elucidates the effect of the injection duration on vascular enhancement: When CM is administered intravenously over a prolonged period of time (say 15–40 s), the arterial enhancement will continuously increase over time, before it decreases rapidly after the end of the injection. One important consequence for CTA is that the general rule that the injection duration equals scanning duration is not universally valid, particularly with faster acquisitions.

The key rules that determine arterial enhancement following an intravenous CM injection in CTA are summarized in Table 1. The derived (user selectable) parameters that control arterial enhancement are therefore:

- *The iodine administration rate.* Vascular enhancement is proportional to the iodine administration rate. Twice the iodine administration rate (for a given injection duration) gives twice the enhancement (and requires twice the CM volume). The iodine administration rate can be varied either by varying the injection flow rate or the concentration of the CM.

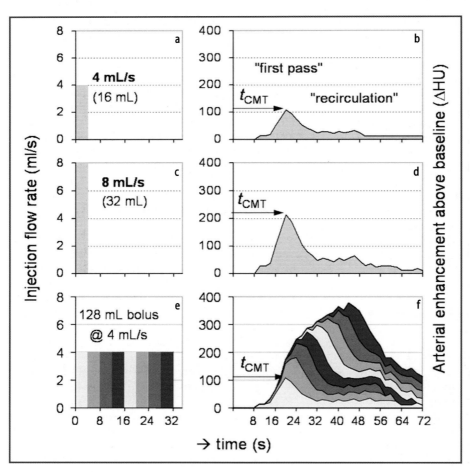

Fig. 1a-f. Relationship between contrast medium (CM) injection and arterial enhancement. Simple "additive model" illustrates the effects of injection flow rate and injection duration on arterial enhancement. Intravenous CM injection (**a**) causes an arterial enhancement response (**b**), which consists of an early "first pass" peak, and a lower "recirculation" effect. Doubling the injection flow rate (doubling the iodine administration rate) (**c**) results in approximately twice the arterial enhancement (**d**). The effect of the injection duration (**e**) can be regarded as the sum (time integral) of several enhancement responses (**f**). Note that due to the asymmetric shape of the test enhancement curve and due to recirculation effects, arterial enhancement following an injection of 128 ml (the "time integral of 8 consecutive 16-ml injections") increases continuously over time (Adapted from [5], with permission)

Table 1. Key rules for arterial enhancement in MDCT

1. Arterial enhancement is proportional to the iodine administration rate (iodine flux), and thus can be contolled by 　• Injection rate (ml / s) 　• Iodine concentration of CM (mg I / ml)
2. Arterial enhancement increases ("cumulative") with prolonged injection duration, and thus can also be controlled by 　• Increasing the scanning delay (relative to CM arrival in the target vessel) and the injection duration
3. An individual's arterial enhancement is inversely related to a patient's cardiac output and central blood volume, both of which are usually unknown, but correlate with body weight 　• Injection volumes and (!) flow rates should be adjusted to body weight [at least for patients with a body weight >90 kg (increase volume and flow rate 20%) and patients with a body weight <60 kg (decrease volume and flow rate 20%)]

CM = contrast medium

– *The injection duration.* Because of recirculation and bolus-broadening effects, longer injection durations lead to continuously increasing and stronger vascular enhancement than shorter injections. Too short injection durations (even with comparably high flow rates) may not reach adequate enhancement levels. Injection durations should be longer than the scanning time with fast acquisitions.

Both the iodine administration rate and the injection duration must be chosen carefully when CTA injection strategies for different scanners and different vascular territories (with different acquisition times) are developed.

Physiological Parameters Affecting Vascular Enhancement

There is a considerable variation between individuals with respect to the degree and time-course of vascular enhancement. For example, the CM transit time (t_{CMT}) from the intravenous injection site to the aorta may vary between 8 and ≥30 s, depending on the injection site and – primarily – on blood flow (cardiac output). Mid-aortic enhancement may range from 140 HU to 440 HU (a factor of 3) between different patients undergoing abdominal CTA [6]. The key physiological parameters affecting individual arterial enhancement are cardiac output and the central blood volume.

Cardiac output is inversely related to the degree of arterial enhancement, particularly in first-pass dynamics [7]. If more blood is ejected per unit of time, the CM injected per unit of time will be more diluted. Hence, arterial enhancement is lower in patients with high cardiac output, but is stronger in patients with low cardiac output (despite the increased t_{CMT} in the latter).

The central blood volume is also inversely related

to arterial enhancement – but presumably affects recirculation and tissue enhancement rather than the first-pass effect [1]. The central blood volume correlates with body weight. However, adjusting the CM dose to body weight will not eliminate the interindividual variability of arterial enhancement [8]; flow rate adjustments for subjects with body weight under 60 kg and over 90 kg are advisable.

Instrumentation and Technique

Power Injectors and Saline Flushing

MDCT generally requires the use of a power injector. Recently, new programmable double-piston power injectors (one syringe for contrast material, one for saline) similar to those used in magnetic resonance angiography have become commercially available. Flushing the venous system with saline immediately after the injection of CM pushes the CM column (approximately 15 ml) from the arm veins, where it may otherwise remain for up to 1 min, into the circulation. Saline flushing improves CM utilization by prolonging and slightly increasing arterial enhancement. Furthermore, it reduces perivenous streak artifacts by removing dense CM from the brachiocephalic veins and the superior vena cava in thoracic and cardiac CT [9].

Accurate Scan Timing Relative to the CM Transit Time t_{CMT}

With faster scanning times, synchronizing the CT acquisition with the desired phase of enhancement is becoming even more critical. With scan times as short as 5–10 s (or less), one may completely miss the bolus if the delay is not properly chosen. Scan timing is individualized according to the respective CM transit time (t_{CMT}). The t_{CMT} can be determined using either a test bolus injection or automatic bolus triggering.

Test Bolus

The injection of a small test bolus (15–20 ml) while acquiring a low-dose dynamic (non-incremental) CT acquisition is a reliable means of determining the t_{CMT} [10]. The t_{CMT} equals the time-to-peak enhancement interval measured from a time-attenuation curve derived from a region of interest (ROI) placed within a reference vessel. The scanning delay of a subsequent full-bolus acquisition is then chosen relative to the t_{CMT}.

Bolus Triggering

Automated bolus triggering is a standard feature of modern MDCT scanners. A ROI is placed into the target vessel on a non-enhanced image. While a full bolus of CM is injected, a series of low-dose non-incremental ("monitoring") images is acquired every 2–3 s, and the enhancement is monitored within ROIs placed in the target vessel. As soon as a predefined enhancement threshold is reached (e.g., 100 HU), the actual MDCT acquisition can be initiated.

While bolus triggering is a clinically useful and robust technique, it is important to be aware of the following technical details: (a) overestimation of the true t_{CMT} inherently occurs due to the sampling rate of the monitoring images; (b) dependent on the scanner type, the image reconstruction time of the monitoring slices may require up to 3 s ("what you see is 3 s old"); and (c) there is a minimum "trigger delay" or "diagnostic delay" needed for preparation of the actual CT acquisition as soon as the threshold is reached. This minimal trigger

delay depends on the scanner model and on the longitudinal distance between the monitoring series and the starting position of the actual CT series (Table 2).

As a practical example, for many four- and eight-channel GE scanner models, the earliest time for initiating an MDCT acquisition is approximately 8 s after the true t_{CMT} (~2 s sampling error plus 3 s image reconstruction time plus 3 s minimum diagnostic delay). Given the previously discussed early CM dynamics, this improves rather than reduces vascular enhancement. However, the relatively delayed acquisition has to be accounted for by increasing the injection duration accordingly (in this example, for 8 s). Otherwise one may run out of CM at the end of the scan. When the properties of a scanner are known and understood, one can use a prolonged scanning delay to advantage (Fig. 2).

CM Concentration

Vascular enhancement (over time) is generally determined by the number of iodine molecules administered (over time). This *iodine administration rate* can therefore be increased either by increasing the injection flow rate and/or by increasing the iodine concentration of the CM used (Table 1). Thus, if one aims at a certain iodine administration rate (e.g., 1.2 g/s), this requires a faster (e.g., 4 ml/s) injection flow rate with standard (300 mg I/ml) CM compared with a slower (e.g., 3 ml/s) flow rate with high-concentration (400 mg I/ml) CM. Very high iodine administration rates, up to 2.4 g/s or more, can be safely injected with a 400 mg I/ml solution at 6 ml/s, whereas an injection flow rate of 8 ml/s would be required using a standard (300 mg I/ml) solution. High iodine administration rates are desirable in CTA, notably in patients with a shallow enhancement response due to an underlying car-

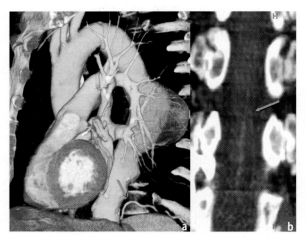

Fig. 2a, b. CTA with increased delay and increased iodine flux for short acquisition time. Volume rendered image (**a**) of a thoracic CT angiogram (16×1.25 mm) obtained in an 84-year-old man with a saccular descending thoracic aortic aneurysm. Adequate opacification is mandatory to identify very small vessels, such as the anterior medullary artery and the great radiculo-medullary artery of Adamkiewicz (*arrow*) in this thin-slab (3-mm) maximum intensity projection image (**b**). The artery of Adamkiewicz is fed by the left 11th intercostals artery (*arrow*). For an acquisition time of only 12 s, a total of 100 ml of CM (350 mg I/ml) was injected at 5 ml/s (injection duration 20 s). The scanning delay was determined using automatic bolus triggering, with initiation of the scan 8 s after CM arriving in the aorta

Table 2. Important facts regarding scan timing with bolus-triggering

- Bolus triggering is generally a robust technique to determine the contrast medium transit time (t_{CMT})

- Bolus triggering inherently delays the start of a CT acquisition, when compared to a test-bolus, because of several factors (sampling rate, image reconstruction time, switching of parameter settings, table movement)

- This inherent delay differs substantially between scanner models

- The inherent delay improves arterial enhancement, but requires an appropriate increase of the injection duration.

diocirculatory disease, and for visualizing very small vessels (Fig. 2). High iodine administration rates are also desirable for non-vascular imaging purposes, e.g., for detecting hypervascular liver lesions or in organ perfusion studies.

Practical Injection Strategies for CTA

Depending on the scanner type, the acquisition parameters, and the vascular territory of interest, MDCT scanning times may vary substantially. Whereas high-resolution acquisitions of large anatomical volumes such as peripheral CTA (Fig. 3) and ECG-gated acquisitions (coronary CTA) have scan times in the order of 30 s, a thoracic CTA may be acquired within 5 s with a 16-channel MDCT scanner. For practical purposes it is therefore useful to (arbitrarily) categorize injection strategies for CTA according to the acquisition time. Long acquisition times benefit from biphasic injections, because they lead to a more favorable uniform enhancement plateau. Fast acquisitions require meticulous scan-timing relative to the t_{CMT} and benefit from high injection (iodine administration) rates.

CM Administration for Slow CTA Acquisitions

When MDCT acquisition times are greater than 15 s, injection durations can be chosen in the traditional way, i.e., equal to the scan time. As a con-

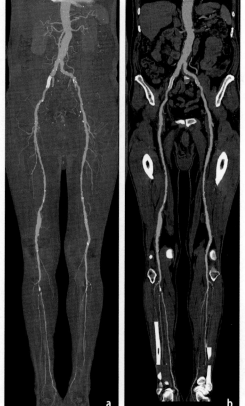

Fig. 3a, b. CTA with biphasic CM injection for prolonged acquisition time. Maximum intensity projection image (**a**) and multi-path curved planar reformation (**b**) of a peripheral CTA data set from a 58-year-old man (16×0.75 mm, 33 s injection duration). Note the patent right external iliac artery stent, the diffuse aneurysmal dilatation of the bilateral popliteal arteries (re>lt) with presumably embolic focal occlusions of the crural arteries. Note the homogeneous arterial opacification of the entire peripheral arterial tree achieved with a biphasic injection using 95 ml of high-concentration CM (400 mg I/ml). The first 25 ml was injected at 4.5 ml/s, the following 70 ml was injected at 2.5 ml/s

tinuous injection of CM leads to a continuous increase of enhancement, vascular opacification will be non-uniform over time, with the brightest enhancement occurring at the end of the acquisition. A more uniform prolonged enhancement can be achieved if biphasic (or multiphasic) injection profiles are employed [3]. Such injections consist of an initial high-rate injection, followed by a longer slow-rate injection phase. Examples are shown in Table 3 and Figure 3. The scanning delay is chosen equal to (or only slightly longer) than the t_{CMT} (t_{CMT} plus 2 s). The minimum trigger delay with Siemens scanners, for example, is currently 2 s.

CM Administration for Fast CTA Acquisitions

Standard injection flow rates (e.g., 4 ml/s of 300 mg I/ml CM) cannot achieve the desired enhancement when the injection duration is too short. To ensure adequate vessel opacification with fast MDCT acquisitions (<15 s), the iodine administration rate needs to be increased if the rule "*injection duration equals scanning duration*" is followed (Table 4). This is achieved either by an increase of the injection flow rate or – more conveniently – by using a higher iodine concentration of the CM. Alternatively, one can also increase the

scanning delay in order to allow the enhancement to increase as well. This strategy is particularly useful for very short acquisition times; however, it requires that the injection duration is also prolonged, which – in return – increases the total CM volume.

Examples of "increased delay protocols" are shown in Table 4 and Figure 1. In this example of a 12-s CTA acquisition, both of the above strategies (increased iodine administration rate and increased delay) are simultaneously applied: For a 12-s CTA acquisition, a delay of t_{CMT} plus 8 s is chosen [this means, the acquisition begins 8 s after the t_{CMT} (a "must" with certain GE scanner models)]. The injection rate is increased to 5 ml/s and a moderately high-concentration contrast agent (350 mg I/ml) used. The injection duration is 20 s (12+8), in order to avoid running out of CM at the end of the scan. This results in a total CM volume of 100 ml (Table 3).

Conclusions

CM-enhanced MDCT has evolved into a powerful imaging modality for non-invasive (minimally invasive) vascular imaging and has replaced diagnostic intra-arterial angiography in many clinical settings. Whereas MDCT technology is continuously evolving, and expanding the diagnostic po-

Table 3. Biphasic Injection Protocols for CTA with 'Long' Acquisition Times

Acquisition time (s)	Scanning delay (s)	Iodine Total dose (g)	Iodine Biphasic iodine flux (g at g/s)	300 mg I/ml CM Total volume (ml)[a]	300 mg I/ml CM Biphasic injections (ml at ml/s)[a]	400 mg I/ml CM Total volume (ml)[b]	400 mg I/ml CM Biphasic injections (ml at ml/s)[b]
40	t_{CMT}+2	42	9 at 1.8 + 33 at 0.95	140	30 at 6 + 110 at 3.1	105	23 at 4.5 + 82 at 2.4
35	t_{CMT}+2	39	9 at 1.8 + 30 at 1.0	130	30 at 6 + 100 at 3.3	100	23 at 4.5 + 77 at 2.5
30	t_{CMT}+2	36	9 at 1.8 + 27 at 1.1	120	30 at 6 + 90 at 3.6	90	23 at 4.5 + 67 at 2.7
25	t_{CMT}+2	33	9 at 1.8 + 24 at 1.2	110	30 at 6 + 80 at 4.0	85	23 at 4.5 + 62 at 3.0
20	t_{CMT}+2	30	9 at 1.8 + 21 at 1.25	100	30 at 6 + 70 at 4.2	75	23 at 4.5 + 52 at 3.1
15	t_{CMT}+2	27	9 at 1.8 + 18 at 1.35	90	30 at 6 + 60 at 4.5	70	23 at 4.5 + 47 at 3.4

t_{CMT} = CM transit time, as established with a test-bolus or bolus-triggering technique
[a] Volume and flow rate calculated for 300 mg I/ml concentration CM
[b] Volume and flow rate calculated for 400 mg I/ml concentration CM

Table 4. Injection protocols for fast CTA acquisitions ("increased delay protocols")

Acquisition time (s)	Scanning delay (s)	Iodine Dose (g)	Iodine flux (g/s)	300 mg I/ml CM CM volume at inj. rate (ml at ml/s)[a]	400 mg I/ml CM CM volume at inj. rate (ml at ml/s)[b]
25	$t_{CMT}+8$	42	1.2	135 at 4.0	100 at 3.0
20	$t_{CMT}+8$	39	1.35	125 at 4.5	95 at 3.4
15	$t_{CMT}+8$	36	1.5	115 at 5	90 at 3.8
10	$t_{CMT}+8$	33	1.8	110 at 6	85 at 4.5
5	$t_{CMT}+10$	27	1.8	90 at 6	70 at 4.5
1	$t_{CMT}+10$	23	1.8	75 at 6	60 at 4.5

t_{CMT} = CM transit time, as established with a test-bolus or bolus-triggering technique
[a] Volume and flow rate calculated for 300 mg I/ml concentration CM
[b] Volume and flow rate calculated for 400 mg I/ml concentration CM

tential of MDCT, it is also becoming more complex, particularly with respect to CM administration. A basic understanding of the physiological and pharmacokinetic principles governing vascular enhancement following an intravenous CM injection will allow us to adapt and optimize injection strategies for current as well as future MDCT applications.

References

1. Dawson P, Blomley MJ (1996) Contrast agent pharmacokinetics revisited. I. Reformulation. Acad Radiology 3[Suppl 2]:S261-S263
2. Fleischmann D, Hittmair K (1999) Mathematical analysis of arterial enhancement and optimization of bolus geometry for CT angiography using the discrete fourier transform. J Comput Assist Tomogr 23:474-484
3. Fleischmann D, Rubin GD, Bankier AA et al (2000) Improved uniformity of aortic enhancement with customized contrast medium injection protocols at CT angiography. Radiology 214:363-371
4. Bae KT, Heiken JP, Brink JA (1998) Aortic and hepatic contrast medium enhancement at CT. I. Prediction with a computer model. Radiology 207:647-655
5. Fleischmann D (2002) Present and future trends in multiple detector-row CT applications: CT angiography. Eur Radiol 12:S11-S16
6. Sheiman RG, Raptopoulos V, Caruso P et al (1996) Comparison of tailored and empiric scan delays for CT angiography of the abdomen. AJR Am J Roentgenol 167:725-729
7. Bae KT, Heiken JP, Brink JA (1998) Aortic and hepatic contrast medium enhancement at CT. II. Effect of reduced cardiac output in a porcine model. Radiology 207:657-662
8. Hittmair K, Fleischmann D (2001) Accuracy of predicting and controlling time-dependent aortic enhancement from a test bolus injection. J Comput Assist Tomogr 25:287-294
9. Haage P, Schmitz-Rode T, Hubner D et al (2000) Reduction of contrast material dose and artifacts by a saline flush using a double power injector in helical CT of the thorax. AJR Am J Roentgenol 174:1049-1053
10. Van Hoe L, Marchal G, Baert AL et al (1995) Determination of scan delay-time in spiral CT-angiography: utility of a test bolus injection. J Comput Assist Tomogr 19:216-220

III.2

Current and Future Indications of Cardiac MDCT

Christoph R. Becker

Introduction

Multidetector-row computed tomography (MDCT) scanners with fast gantry rotation and simultaneous acquisition of an electrocardiogram (ECG) allow for investigations with high spatial and temporal resolution mandatory for the heart and coronary arteries. The scan mode dedicated to cardiac MDCT is called retrospective ECG gating [1]. For this technique the spiral CT scan is acquired with a slow table feed and image reconstruction is performed in the slow-motion diastole phase of the cardiac cycle.

Cardiac MDCT can be applied for coronary calcium screening and plaque imaging, coronary CT angiography (CTA), and assessment of myocardial function. Different scan protocols exist for various clinical questions. Coronary calcium screening requires investigation of the entire heart without contrast medium and with 3-mm slices. Overlapping slice reconstruction improves reproducibility of the coronary calcium quantification [2]. As a fundamental requirement for screening, the radiation exposure for coronary calcium scanning is reduced to a minimum (approximately 2 mSv). ECG pulsing allows for further reduction by 50% of the redundant exposure occurring during systole [3].

Coronary CTA for plaque imaging and detection of coronary artery stenoses requires the highest temporal and spatial resolution. Depending on the technical possibilities, scan and contrast protocols are different for every MDCT scanner (Table 1).

Current Clinical Applications

Coronary Calcium Screening

Coronary atherosclerosis begins as early as the 1st decade of life with endothelia dysfunction, proliferation of smooth muscle cells, and accumulation of fat (fatty streaks) in the coronary artery wall [4]. During the later stage of the disease, these lesions may further accumulate cholesterol within the intimal and media layer of the coronary artery wall, with a fibrous cap separating the lipid pool from the coronary artery lumen [5]. Inflammatory processes with invasion of macrophages and activation of matrix metalloproteases cause consecutive weakening of the fibrous cap [6]. This vulnerable plaque may rupture when exposed to shear stress and its thrombogenic lipid material may enter the bloodstream. In the worst scenario, thrombus progression may turn the vulnerable plaque

Table 1. Scan and contrast parameters for coronary CTA

	4-detector CT	16-detector CT	64-detector CT
Collimation	4×1 mm	16×0.75 mm	[a]2×32×0.6 mm
Gantry rotation	500 ms	420–370[b] ms	330 ms
Scan time	~40 s	~20 s	~10 s
Iomeprol (Iomeron 400)	80/60[c] ml	80 ml	40 ml
Flow	4/3[c] ml/s	4 ml/s	4 ml/s

[a]Dual z-focus
[b]With Straton tube
[c]First/second phase

into a culprit lesion that occludes the coronary vessel, leading to myocardial ischemia, ventricular fibrillation, and death [7].

In many patients, unheralded myocardial infarction associated with a mortality of approximately 20% is the first sign of coronary artery disease (CAD). The risk of an event strongly depends on risk factors, such as hypertension, hypercholesteremia, smoking habits, family history, age, and gender. Based of these risk factors, the Framingham [8] and PROCAM [9] algorithms provide an estimation of the midterm (10-year) risk for an individual subject to experience a cardiac event. According to international guidelines, subjects with a midterm risk of less than 10% are considered to be at low risk and usually do not require any specific therapy. Patients with a midterm risk of more than 20% are considered to be at high risk and therefore may also be called subjects with a CAD equivalent. Similar to patients with established CAD, these asymptomatic subjects may require intensive therapy, such as lifestyle changes and lifetime medical treatment.

Approximately 40% of the population is considered to have a moderate midterm risk of 10%–20%. All of the stratification schemes suffer from a lack of accuracy in correctly determining the risk, and uncertainty exists as to how to treat subjects who have been identified to be at intermediate risk. Other tools providing information about the necessity to either reassure or to treat these subjects are warranted. Currently, assessment of the atherosclerotic plaque burden is considered to provide valid information for this cohort [10].

Arad et al. were the first to report attempts to predict cardiac events with coronary calcium as detected by electron beam CT (EBCT). The calcifications were quantified according to the algorithm of Agatston et al. [11]. In their cohort of 1,173 patients, they observed 26 soft (PTCA and bypass grafting) and hard (myocardial infarction and death) events over a period of 19 months. If the Agatston score was above 160 the odds ratio for an event was 20–35.4. Raggi et al. [12] used age- and gender-specific percentiles derived from nearly 10,000 patients to identify patients at increased risk for an event; 70% of patients with an unheralded myocardial infarction ($n=172$) had a calcium score above the 75th percentile compared with an asymptomatic cohort ($n=632$).

One of the major limitations of the Agatston score is its low reproducibility [13]. Callister et al. [14] introduced the volume equivalent with isotropic interpolation for improved reproducibility. With this quantification algorithm they were able to determine the progression rates of coronary calcium in patients with hypercholesterolemia under statin therapy. Untreated patients with a low-density lipoprotein (LDL) level of over 120 mg/dl had an annual calcium volume progression of 52%. Patients treated with statins with an LDL level above and below 120 mg/dl had an annual progression rate of 25% and –7%, respectively [15]. Although other authors have confirmed this observation, it is as yet unclear how the changes of the calcified plaque burden affect the cardiac event risk.

Because of different acquisition mode and image quality, the Agatston score and volume equivalent are not comparable and reproducible between EBCT and MDCT. An international consortium of all CT vendors (Siemens, Toshiba, Philips, General Electric) and some leading research and clinical institutions has recently agreed upon a standardized measurement for coronary calcium. The consortium provides guidelines for standardized CT scan protocols for any company, as well as guidelines for calibration, quantification, and quality assurance. In addition, the consortium has agreed upon the absolute mass quantification as the algorithm with the highest inter-scanner reproducibility. Once finalized, the consortium will also provide a web-based database entry allowing estimation of the event risk based on Framingham, PROCAM, and other algorithms, as well as for age- and gender-specific percentile ranking of the calcium mass [16].

Currently, all these strategies provide two different numbers for the risk according to the conventional risk assessment and the amount of coronary calcium. It has recently been reported that the combined use of the Framingham risk assessment and the calcium measurement is superior to the selected use of the Framingham risk assessment alone [17]. The weak point of the Framingham risk algorithm is that higher age becomes the predominant factor above all others. This assumption certainly does not fit all subjects. Therefore, Grundy [18] proposed an alternative scheme in which the age score in Framingham is replaced by a scheme that takes into account the coronary calcium percentiles. If the amount of coronary calcium is between the 25th and 75th percentiles, the Framingham risk score remains unchanged. If the amount of calcium is below the 25th or above the 75th percentile, the score is the same as for subjects approximately 10 years younger or older, respectively.

Coronary CTA

Contrast-enhanced CTA of the coronary arteries is a new application of MDCT. Coronary artery enhancement mainly depends on the contrast medium density and injection rate [19]. With shorter scan times, as with the 16- and 64-detector row CT scanners, a mono-phase bolus of 80 and 40 ml

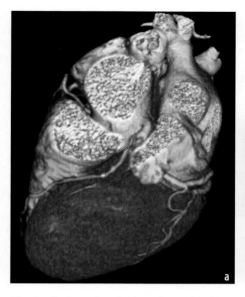
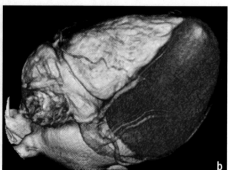

Fig. 1a, b. Several studies have shown that the negative predictive value of CTA is approximately 98%. CTA investigation of an 80-year-old woman with left branch block with the suspicion of coronary artery disease. All coronary segments are well assessable and no stenoses or atherosclerosis can be detected. The left branch block in this patient is most likely due to cardiomyopathy

Iomeprol (Iomeron 400) may be administered, respectively. With longer scan times, as for the four-detector-row CT, a dual-phase contrast protocol is required to compensate for contrast recirculation in the later phase of the injection and to maintain constant and homogeneous enhancement of approximately 300 HU for the entire scan range (Table 1). Iomeprol should always be administered at body temperature (37°C).

The use of a dual-head injector for the sequential injection of contrast medium and saline is mandatory to keep the contrast bolus compact. In MDCT scanners with shorter scan times, a saline chaser bolus also results in a wash-out of contrast medium from the right ventricle, helping to reduce artifacts caused by the influx of undiluted contrast medium from the superior vena cava [20].

First reports comparing coronary CTA and conventional catheter-based coronary angiography for the detection of coronary artery stenoses were encouraging [21-23]. In particular, for the 16-detector row CT, sensitivity and specificity values between 86% and 95% have been reported [24, 25]. However, such high values can only be achieved if non-evaluable coronary segments are excluded from analysis. In fact, most of the coronary segments were excluded because of motion artifacts. Motion-free images have only been achieved in patients with low and regular heart rates. The administration of metoprolol (Beloc) at the start of the investigation may help to reduce the heart rate and hence improve the image quality.

One of the other limitations in the detection of stenoses and plaques with coronary MDCT angiography is related to calcium or any other dense material such as metallic stents. These components are exaggerated by CT and prevent assessment of the coronary artery wall and lumen. For this reason, patients with chronic stable angina who may have extensive calcifications or patients after coronary stent placement should currently not be considered for a CTA investigation.

However, coronary CTA has a high negative predictive value compared with cardiac catheterization. In patients with non-specific complaints or ambiguous stress tests, CTA may serve as a reliable non-invasive alternative to rule out CAD (Fig. 1).

Coronary CTA is also well suited to visualize the anatomy in patients with coronary anomalies and to identify patients in whom the aberrant coronary artery has its course in between the ascending aorta and the pulmonary outflow tract. In this particular location the coronary artery is at risk of being squeezed between the two major vessels, which may subsequently result in myocardial ischemia. Coronary CTA may also provide valid and useful information in patients with vasculitis and aneurysms [26], fistulas (Fig. 2), or dissection.

In addition to displaying the contrast-filled lumen like cardiac catheterization, CTA as a cross-sectional modality can also display the coronary artery wall. Coronary atherosclerotic changes may appear as calcified, non-calcified, or mixed plaques. In a recently published study, Leber et al. [27] reported that non-calcified lesions were predominantly found in patients with acute myocardial infarction, whereas calcified lesions were

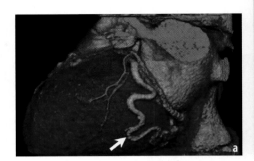

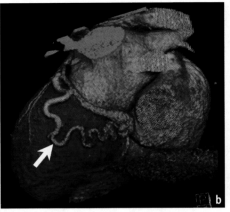

Fig. 2a, b. Patient with a heart murmur. The CTA investigation demonstrates a fistula of the circumflex coronary artery (*arrow*) with kinking draining into the right atrium

found more often in patients with chronic stable angina. In patients with an acute coronary syndrome, a non-calcified lesion in the coronary artery may correspond to an intra coronary thrombus [28] (Fig. 3).

The current gold standard for the detection of coronary atherosclerosis in vivo is intravascular ultrasonography (IVUS). Studies comparing IVUS with MDCT have shown a good correlation between the echogeneity and CT density of coronary atherosclerotic lesions [29]. The sensitivity and specificity of CT for the detection of calcified and non-calcified coronary atherosclerosis is 78% and 94%, respectively. However, the sensitivity for the detection of non-calcified plaques in a lesion-by-lesion comparison of CTA and IVUS was only 52% [30].

CT density measurement in carotid arteries [31] and heart specimens [32] has shown that CT densities of 50 HU and 90 HU within plaques are specific for lipid and fibrous tissue, respectively. In a recent study by Langheinrich et al. [33] with micro-CT and ultrahigh spatial resolution, the ability of CT to distinguish between different plaque components such as lipid, fibrin, and calcium was demonstrated. Interestingly, the proliferation of smooth muscle cells also increases the CT density of the plaque.

Recently, we observed a plaque in a patient with unstable angina who developed a myocardial infarction in due course with a culprit lesion at the location of the former plaque. The vulnerable plaque that had been detected prior to its rupture had a dark center surrounded by a bright rim, most likely corresponding to a lipid pool and a fibrous cap, respectively (Fig. 4).

Future Technical and Clinical Potential

Current ongoing prospective cohort studies such as the PACC [34], RECALL [35], and MESA [36] studies will determine the predictive value of coronary calcium for cardiac events. If the results, expected by the end of this decade, are positive, coronary calcium percentile ranking in combination with conventional risk assessment will be incorporated in future prevention guidelines.

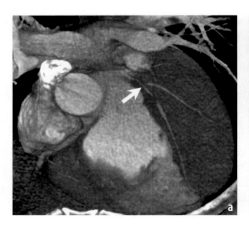

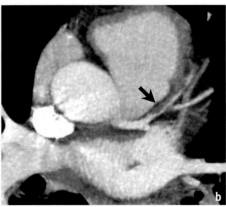

Fig. 3a, b. Images of a patient with acute myocardial infarction. Volume rendering of the CTA data set (**a**) demonstrates a high-grade stenosis (*arrow*). The maximum intensity image (**b**) demonstrates the culprit lesion in the corresponding location (*arrow*) most likely corresponding to thrombus formation (low CT densities and irregular borders)

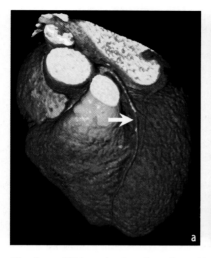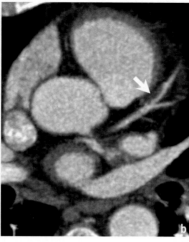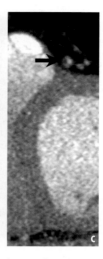

Fig. 4a-c. CTA investigation of a patient with unstable angina without signs of myocardial ischemia. The volume rendering of the data set (**a**) shows a regular vessel lumen. The axial slice (**b**), however, demonstrates a well-defined plaque in the middle segment of the left anterior descending coronary artery (*arrow*). The perpendicular reformatting (**c**) demonstrates a vulnerable plaque with a low dense (fatty) center surrounded by high-density (fibrous) tissue. In due course (3 weeks later) this plaque ruptured, resulting in an anterior wall infarction in this patient

With the standardization of coronary calcium measurements, the results of these studies, originally obtained with EBCT, may be transferred to MDCT. MDCT scanners are already widely available and therefore will allow for widespread use of coronary calcium scanning for further risk stratification in subjects with an intermediate cardiac event risk.

If CTA can detect vulnerable plaques in patients with acute coronary syndrome directly, new strategies need to be considered for appropriate treatment of these patients. The detection of noninvasive vulnerable plaques may justify intensive medical treatment or may lead to invasive approaches such as plaque sealing.

In patients with atypical chest pain, CTA may soon serve as a tool for the complete diagnostic work-up of patients. A single CTA investigation will allow detection of pulmonary emboli, aortic dissection, or coronary thrombus. Currently, however, it appears unlikely that coronary CTA will be used as a screening tool for vulnerable plaques in asymptomatic subjects because of the necessity to administer contrast medium and the comparatively high radiation exposure of this application.

Some technical improvements of MDCT are foreseen within the next few years; these include shorter exposure times and higher spatial resolution. Exposure times will become short enough to scan the coronary arteries at any heart rate without the necessity to administer beta-blockers, and the higher spatial resolution will reduce the artifact caused by metal or calcium. Once these requirements are fulfilled, coronary CTA may replace cardiac catheterization for the triage of patients for conservative, interventional, or surgical therapy and may restrict the use of an invasive diagnostic procedure to pre-selected patients in whom coronary interventions are essential.

References

1. Flohr T, Ohnesorge B (2001) Heart rate adaptive optimization of spatial and temporal resolution for electrocardiogram-gated multislice spiral CT of the heart. J Comput Assist Tomogr 25:907-923
2. Ohnesorge B, Flohr T, Fischbach R et al (2002) Reproducibility of coronary calcium quantification in repeat examinations with retrospectively ECG-gated multisection spiral CT. Eur Radiol 12:1532-1540
3. Jakobs TF, Becker CR, Ohnesorge B et al (2002) Multislice helical CT of the heart with retrospective ECG gating: reduction of radiation exposure by ECG-controlled tube current modulation. Eur Radiol 12:1081-1086
4. Stary HC, Chandler AB, Glagov S et al (1994) A definition of initial, fatty streak, and intermediate lesions of atherosclerosis. A report from the Committee on Vascular Lesions of the Council on Arteriosclerosis, American Heart Association. Circulation 89:2462-2478
5. Stary HC, Chandler AB, Dinsmore RE et al (1995) A definition of advanced types of atherosclerotic lesions and a histological classification of atherosclerosis. A report from the Committee on Vascular Lesions of the Council on Arteriosclerosis, American Heart Association. Circulation 92:1355-1374
6. Pasterkamp G, Falk E, Woutman H et al (2000) Techniques characterizing the coronary atherosclerotic plaque: influence on clinical decision making? J Am Coll Cardiol 36:13-21
7. Virmani R, Kolodgie FD, Burke AP et al (2000)

Lessons from sudden coronary death. A comprehensive morphological classification scheme for atherosclerotic lesions. Arterioscler Thromb Vasc Biol 20:1262-1275

8. Wilson PW, D'Agostino RB, Levy D et al (1998) Prediction of coronary heart disease using risk factor categories. Circulation 97:1837-1847

9. Assmann G, Cullen P, Schulte H (2002) Simple scoring scheme for calculating the risk of acute coronary events based on the 10-year follow-up of the prospective cardiovascular Munster (PROCAM) study. Circulation 105:310-315

10. Greenland P, Abrams J, Aurigemma GP et al (2000) Prevention Conference V: beyond secondary prevention: identifying the high-risk patient for primary prevention: noninvasive tests of atherosclerotic burden: Writing Group III. Circulation 101:E16-E22

11. Agatston AS, Janowitz WR, Hildner FJ et al (1990) Quantification of coronary artery calcium using ultrafast computed tomography. J Am Coll Cardiol 15:827-832

12. Raggi P, Callister TQ, Cooil B et al (2000) Identification of patients at increased risk of first unheralded acute myocardial infarction by electron-beam computed tomography. Circulation 101:850-855

13. Hernigou A, Challande P, Boudeville JC et al (1996) Reproducibility of coronary calcification detection with electron-beam computed tomography. Eur Radiol 6:210-216

14. Callister TQ, Cooil B, Raya SP et al (1998) Coronary artery disease: improved reproducibility of calcium scoring with an electron-beam CT volumetric method. Radiology 208:807-814

15. Callister T, Janowitz W, Raggi P (2000) Sensitivity of two electron beam tomography protocols for the detection and quantification of coronary artery calcium. AJR Am J Radiol 175:1743-1746

16. McCollough CH, Ulzheimer S, Halliburton SS et al (2003) A multi-scanner, multi-manufacturer, international standard for the quantification of coronary artery calcium using cardiac CT. Radiology 229:630

17. Greenland P, LaBree L, Azen SP et al (2004) Coronary artery calcium score combined with Framingham score for risk prediction in asymptomatic individuals. JAMA 291:210-215

18. Grundy SM (2001) Coronary plaque as a replacement for age as a risk factor in global risk assessment. AJR Am J Cardiol 88:8E-11E

19. Becker CR, Hong C, Knez A et al (2003) Optimal contrast application for cardiac 4-detector-row computed tomography. Invest Radiol 38:690-694

20. Cademartiri F, Mollet N, Lugt A van der et al (2004) Non-invasive 16-row multislice CT coronary angiography: usefulness of saline chaser. Eur Radiol 14:178-183

21. Achenbach S, Giesler T, Ropers D et al (2001) Detection of coronary artery stenoses by contrast-enhanced, retrospectively electrocardiographically-gated, multislice spiral computed tomography. Circulation 103:2535-2538

22. Nieman K, Oudkerk M, Rensing B et al (2001) Coronary angiography with multi-slice computed computed tomography. Lancet 357:599-603

23. Knez A, Becker CR, Leber A et al (2001) Usefulness of multislice spiral computed tomography angiography for determination of coronary artery stenoses. AJR Am J Cardiol 88:1191-1194

24. Nieman K, Cademartiri F, Lemos PA et al (2002) Reliable noninvasive coronary angiography with fast submillimeter multislice spiral computed tomography. Circulation 106:2051-2054

25. Ropers D, Baum U, Pohle K et al (2003) Detection of coronary artery stenoses with thin-slice multi-detector row spiral computed tomography and multiplanar reconstruction. Circulation 107:664-666

26. Fallenberg M, Juergens KU, Wichter T et al (2002) Coronary artery aneurysm and type-A aortic dissection demonstrated by retrospectively ECG-gated multislice spiral CT. Eur Radiol 12:201-204

27. Leber AW, Knez A, White CW et al (2003) Composition of coronary atherosclerotic plaques in patients with acute myocardial infarction and stable angina pectoris determined by contrast-enhanced multislice computed tomography. AJR Am J Cardiol 91:714-718

28. Becker CR, Knez A, Ohnesorge B et al (2000) Imaging of noncalcified coronary plaques using helical CT with retrospective ECG gating. AJR Am J Roentgenol 175:423-424

29. Schroeder S, Kopp AF, Baumbach A et al (2001) Noninvasive detection of coronary lesions by multislice computed tomography: results of the New Age pilot trial. Catheter Cardiovasc Interv 53:352-358

30. Achenbach S, Moselewski F, Ropers D et al (2004) Detection of calcified and noncalcified coronary atherosclerotic plaque by contrast-enhanced, submillimeter multidetector spiral computed tomography: a segment-based comparison with intravascular ultrasound. Circulation 109:14-17

31. Estes J, Quist W, Lo Gerfo F et al (1998) Noninvasive characterization of plaque morphology using helical computed tomography. J Cardiovasc Surg 39:527-534

32. Becker CR, Nikolaou K, Muders M et al (2003) Ex vivo coronary atherosclerotic plaque characterization with multi-detector-row CT. Eur Radiol 13:2094-2098

33. Langheinrich AC, Bohle RM, Greschus S et al (2004) Atherosclerotic lesions at micro CT: feasibility for analysis of coronary artery wall in autopsy specimens. Radiology 231:675-681

34. O´Malley P, Taylor A, Gibbons R et al (1999) Rationale and design of the prospective army coronary calcium (PACC) study: utility of electron beam computed tomography as a screening test for coronary artery disease and as an intervention for risk factor modification among young, asymptomatic, active-duty United States Army personel. Am Heart J 137:932-941

35. Schmermund A, Mohlenkamp S, Stang A et al (2002) Assessment of clinically silent atherosclerotic disease and established and novel risk factors for predicting myocardial infarction and cardiac death in healthy middle-aged subjects: rationale and design of the Heinz Nixdorf RECALL Study. Risk Factors, Evaluation of Coronary Calcium and Lifestyle. Am Heart J 144:212-218

36. National Heart, Lung and Blood Institute (2000) NHLBI launches 10-year study on early detection of heart disease. Accessed at http://www.nhlbi.nih.gov/new/press/sep14-00.htm

III.3

Abdominal Aorta, Renal Arteries and Run-Off Vessels

Carlo Catalano, Alessandro Napoli, Francesco Fraioli, Mario Cavacece,
Linda Bertoletti, Piergiorgio Nardis and Roberto Passariello

Introduction

After the introduction of spiral computed tomography (CT), there was a dramatic increase in the clinical indications for CT angiography (CTA), with a large number of studies performed worldwide, especially after the development of multidetector-row CT (MDCT) technology. MDCT allows the simultaneous acquisition of four or more (the number is continuously increasing) slices per single gantry rotation with a speed at least eight times that of single-slice spiral CT, as well as excellent longitudinal resolution and near-isotropic voxels. MDCT has had a significant effect on CTA by enabling high spatial resolution even when imaging large volumes, with excellent visualization of small branches after a single bolus administration of contrast agent [1-3]. As a result, CTA has become a valid method for diagnostic vascular imaging, challenging digital subtraction angiography (DSA) in most areas. DSA is now performed only as a first step during interventional procedures.

Indications for vascular imaging of the abdominal aorta, renal arteries, and lower extremity arteries include peripheral atherosclerotic arterial disease (PAD), aneurysm, vasculitis, vascular masses, and trauma. PAD more commonly affects the renal arteries and lower extremities, causing symptoms that range from nephro-vascular hypertension to intermittent claudication and/or limb-threatening ischemia.

Lesions can be distinguished by type (atheromatous versus thromboembolic), chronicity (acute versus chronic), severity (mild, moderate, severe stenosis), length (focal, short, long segment), vessel wall location (circumferential versus eccentric), and vascular territory (inflow versus outflow).

In most cases, aneurysm affects the abdominal aorta, although wall dilatation can be seen in any vascular segment of the body, including the renal and run-off arteries (especially the popliteal arteries, Fig. 1). Vasculitis more frequently affects the upper extremities. Systemic symptoms are not uncommon; patients may present with a combination of claudication, rest ischemia, and/or Raynaud's

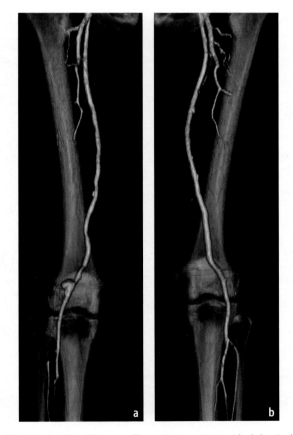

Fig. 1a, b. CTA of the run-off vessels in a patient with abdominal aortic aneurysm (AAA, not shown in the figure) with a left popliteal pulsating mass (popliteal aneurysm); **a** and **b** show left leg and right leg respectively, back view. Both images are reformatted with a volume rendering (VR) technique that allows a prospective view. In both cases bony editing has been performed, and bones have been subsequently displayed on the transparency, giving excellent anatomical boundary

phenomenon, depending on the disease burden, level of involvement, and collateral flow. Vascular masses include aneurysms, hemangiomas, and arterio venous malformations. Both acute and chronic vascular injuries can be easily and successfully evaluated with CTA.

Key factors for successful CTA include the combination of the best scanning profile with the precise delivery of the contrast medium, as well as high-quality imaging display by means of multiple three-dimensional reformations. A detailed description of the current CTA scanning protocols, contrast medium administration strategies, and

three-dimensional image reconstruction approaches for the renal arteries, abdominal aorta, and run-off vessels ensues.

Scanning Protocol

The scanning profile employed for CTA of the renal arteries as well as the infrarenal abdominal aorta and run-off arteries largely depends on the scanner type available (4-, 8-, 16-, or 64-row). Scanning protocols with different CT scanners and detector technology are summarized in Tables 1-3.

Table 1. Acquisition parameters for four-channel MDCT units

Acquisition	Manufacturers	Detector configuration (channels×mm)	Pitch	Table speed (mm/s)	Scan time (s)[a]
Fast volume coverage	GE	4×2.5	1.5	18.75	16
	Philips	4×2.5	1.5	30	10
	Siemens	4×2.5	1.5	30	10
	Toshiba	4×2	1.375	22	14
High-resolution	GE	4×1.25	1.5	9.375	32
	Philips	4×1	1.5	12	25
	Siemens	4×1	1.5	12	25
	Toshiba	4×1	1.375	11	27
Submillimeter-isotropic resolution	GE)	2×0.625	1.5	2.3	65
	Philips	2×0.5	0.8	1.6	94
	Siemens	2×0.5	0.8	1.6	94
	Toshiba	4×0.5	0.75	3	50

[a]Scan time for hypothetic volume coverage of 30 cm

Table 2. Acquisition parameters for eight-channel MDCT units

Acquisition	Manufacturers	Detector configuration (channels×mm)	Pitch	Table speed (mm/s)	Scan time (s)[a]
Fast volume coverage	GE	8×2.5	1.35	54	5.5
High-resolution	GE	8×1.25	1.5	27	11.1
Submillimeter-isotropic resolution	GE	2×0.625	1.5	2.3	65.22

[a]Scan time for hypothetic volume coverage of 30 cm

Table 3. Acquisition parameters for 16-channel MDCT units

Acquisition	Manufacturers	Detector configuration (channels×mm)	Pitch	Table speed (mm/s)	Scan time (s)[a]
High-resolution	GE	16×1.25	1.375	55	5.5
	Philips	16×1.5	1.25	60	5
	Siemens	16×1.5	1.5	72	4
	Toshiba	16×2	0.9375	60	5
Submillimeter-isotropic resolution	GE)	16×0.625	1.375	27.5	11
	Philips	16×0.75	1.25	30	10
	Siemens	16×0.75	1.5	43	7
	Toshiba	16×0.5	1.4375	23	13

[a]Scan time for hypothetic volume coverage of 30 cm

Renal Arteries

To assess abnormalities of the renal arteries, the patient is placed head-first and supine on the scanner table, and is then asked to hold his/her breath during the scanning procedure. As for regular examinations of the abdomen, an initial topogram (512 mm) is obtained from the diaphragm to the pelvis in order to correctly place the acquisition volume on the kidney area.

Scanning prior to the administration of contrast medium is not routinely performed for CTA, but is not an option when looking for lithiasis or hemorrhage, such as intralesional bleeding (i.e., angiomyolypoma). Due to the relatively small anatomical volume to be examined, the renal arteries are usually scanned using a high-resolution protocol, regardless of the number of simultaneous helices acquired with the existing CT scanner (4-, 8-, or 16-row). A near-isotropic to submillimeter (1.25–0.75 mm) detector configuration is always employed for excellent arterial detail. Even with a detector configuration of 4×1 mm, which virtually represents the slowest scan configuration achievable with an MDCT scanner, the scan time is reasonably short, allowing scanning within a single breath hold at the highest in-plane resolution.

Abdominal Aorta and Run-Off Arteries

The patient is placed feet-first and supine on the scanner table. The legs are secured with cushions and adhesive tape as close to the isocenter of the scanner as possible. In order to separate the tibia from the fibula, and consequently the trifurcation vessels from the bones, the patient's feet can be tied at a slight degree of internal rotation. This trick, although not in universal use, can facilitate post-processing and more easily display the calf vessels. A large topogram (1,024 mm) is obtained from the diaphragm to the feet in order to position the acquisition volume and examine the arterial district from the celiac trunk to the pedal circulation [6].

Using a 4-channel MDCT scanner with a gantry rotation time of 0.5 s, the following protocol has proved successful: 4×2.5-mm collimation, 3-mm section thickness, 50% slice overlap, table feed of 15 mm per gantry rotation (30 mm/s), resulting in a scan time between 35 and 45 s, depending on the patient length. With a 4-channel MDCT scanner, 3-mm slice thickness yields a relatively thin slice in a sufficiently fast mode. Thin-section acquisitions (~1 mm) provide excellent detail but are limited by image noise (abdomen), long scan times, and as a consequence by venous opacification, especially in the lower limbs.

Protocols for 8-channel MDCT scanners are: 8×1.25-mm collimation, a table feed of 16.75 mm per gantry rotation (33.5 mm/s), resulting in a scan time between 31 and 39 s, or 8×2.5-mm collimation, a table feed of 33.5 mm per gantry rotation (67 mm/s) with a scanning time between 16 and 20 s.

Protocols for 16-channel MDCT depend on the detector configuration and scanner. With 16-channel MDCT scanners, either high- or low-resolution protocols can be successfully used, without any risk of venous contamination or excessively slow scanning. A high-resolution protocol can be performed using a collimation between 16×0.75-mm and 16×0.63-mm, depending on the manufacturer, with a similar table feed of 17.5–18 mm/rotation and a scanning time between 29 and 37 s.

Lower-resolution protocols can also be utilized, reducing the scan time: 16×1.25–1.5-mm collima-

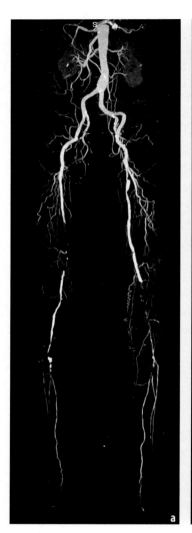
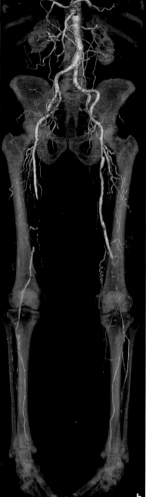
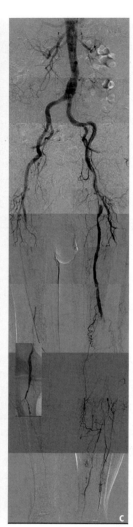

Fig. 2a-c. Patient with bilateral rest pain and critical limb ischemia. CTA studies reformatted with maximum intensity projection (MIP) (**a**) and VR (**b**) technique show diffuse atherosclerotic changes of the run-off district, with occlusion of the right superficial femoral artery (SFA), dilatation of the right popliteal artery, multiple stenotic lesions of the left SFA, occlusion of its distal portion, and extensive arterial collateral net visualization, as confirmed by digital subtraction angiography (DSA) (**c**)

tion, table feed of 33–35 mm per gantry rotation, and a scanning time between 15 and 20 s. Compared with 4-channel MDCT, 8-channel MDCT affords greater temporal resolution, while 16-channel MDCT affords both greater temporal and spatial resolution. When compared with 4-channel MDCT, for the same volume coverage, collimation, gantry rotation, and nominal section thickness, scan times are twice as fast with 8-channel MDCT and 4 times faster with 16-channel MDCT. When using 16-channel MDCT, thinner sections can be obtained (0.625 mm) with still half the scan time of four-channel MDCT. The thinner acquisition (≤1.25 mm) provides high-resolution isotropic data sets, which improve image quality and three-dimensional post-processing.

In contrast to other vascular areas, such as the coronaries, even 4-channel MDCT scanners provide excellent results in the evaluation of PAD (Fig. 2), as shown by all articles published to date on the topic.

In most cases, whenever performing CTA of the abdominal aorta and run-off arteries, the kidney area is included in the scanned volume. Therefore renal arteries (small volume) are acquired with the regular scan protocol as per the run-off arteries (large volume). However, renal arteries are smaller in caliber than most arteries of the run-off vasculature and may be poorly seen without further processing. In general, as we cannot modify the scan protocol, we tend to reconstruct the entire volume with a relatively large image thickness (3 mm, reconstruction interval 3 mm) and to produce a second volume, targeted to the renal arteries using reconstruction with a thinner interval (3 mm, 1-mm reconstruction interval).

Image Reconstruction

Standard-resolution CTA data sets can be obtained from 2.5- to 3-mm MDCT acquisitions, whereby

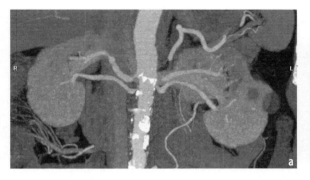
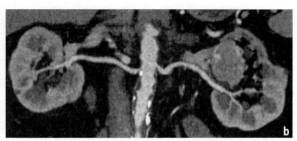

Fig. 3a, b. CTA performed with a standard fast scan protocol for run-off arteries (4×3 mm) and subsequently reconstructed with a thinner reconstruction interval (1 mm) of the kidney area. The MIP (**a**) image clearly shows bilateral double renal arteries. Atherosclerotic changes are seen on all four arteries and are better visualized with a curved planar reconstruction (**b**) along the course of the arteries

overlapping images are reconstructed every 1- to 1.5-mm. Depending on the existing image storage capabilities, for a large volume it may be preferable to reconstruct the entire volume with relatively large intervals (2.5–3 mm). Manufacturers allow further reconstruction of the scanned volume with a thinner interval (0.5–1 mm) for selected areas. This is especially important when examining the inflow and run-off district, which is a large arterial volume generating a proportionately large number of images. Therefore, thinner reconstruction can be performed on a second reconstruction task targeted to the kidney area for fine depiction of the renal arteries, thus limiting the number of images created (Fig. 3).

High-resolution isotropic data sets can be obtained from thin collimation (≤1.25 mm) acquisition, whereby overlapping images are reconstructed at 0.5- to 0.8-mm increments. Thinner reconstructions produce higher image quality for depicting small vessels, but require greater processing speed and archival storage to deal with the larger volume of data. Furthermore, the thin-section data sets are limited by increased image noise in the abdomen, requiring increased milliamperes.

Contrast Agent Administration

Abdominal Aorta and Run-Off Arteries

The administration of the bolus of contrast agent is crucial for the successful performance of peripheral CTA. The aim of a CTA study is to obtain a constant enhancement of arterial structures, even of small caliber, throughout the acquisition, without venous contamination. It must be borne in mind that the best contrast enhancement in CT is obtained when the maximum concentration of iodine in the scanned volume is reached during the effective acquisition temporal window.

Optimization of contrast medium administra-tion is the key factor for achieving a good peripheral MDCT vascular examination, particularly in patients with peripheral arterial occlusive disease (PAD), and especially with faster (8- and 16-channel) scanners. The flow rate, iodine concentration, amount of contrast agent, and delay time all affect the image quality.

The contrast medium transit time from the injection site to the beginning of the scan volume varies for individual patients. In 95% of patients the time between the injection of contrast agent and its arrival at the abdominal aorta ranges between 14 and 28 s. To account for this variability, scan delays should be individualized. This can be accomplished by calculation of the delay time, either with a test bolus or an automated bolus-triggering technique.

Because many patients with PAD may have co-existing cardiovascular disease with reduced cardiac output, initial enhancement profiles may be shallow. In this case, an increase of the initial injection flow rate (e.g., 5–6 ml/s for the first 5 s of the injection), use of a high-concentration contrast medium (≥350–400 mg I/ml), or an increased scanning delay relative to the contrast arrival in the aorta (i.e., 8 s) are options for eliminating this problem.

In patients with PAD, flow-limiting arterial stenoses and occlusions may be present anywhere between the infrarenal aorta and the pedal arteries in the leg. The bolus transit time from the aorta to the popliteal arteries, for example, ranged from 4 to 24 s (mean 10 s) in a group of 20 patients with PAD. The clinical stage of the disease was no predictor of aorto-popliteal bolus transit time. Extrapolated for the entire peripheral arterial tree and across individuals, an injection duration of 35 s is necessary to guarantee optimal opacification of the aorta down to the pedal branches in all (>97.5%) patients. With 4-channel MDCT this is not relevant, because acquisition times are usually longer than 35 s. With 8- and 16-channel scanners, however, the CT acquisition may outrun the bolus

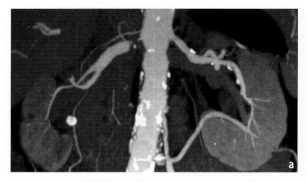

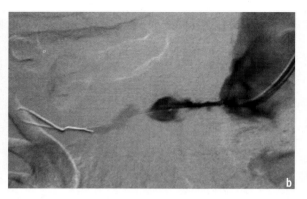

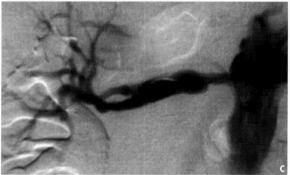

Fig. 4a-c. Patient with nephro-vascular hypertension. CTA with MIP (**a**) reconstruction shows right renal artery stenosis and post-stenotic dilation of the artery, which also presents early bifurcation. DSA, performed subsequently, confirmed the tight stenotic lesion (**b**) and allowed treatment maneuvers (**c**)

if the scanning protocol does not account for possible slow arterial filling.

In the case of asymmetric flow, differences in enhancement of the two extremities may occur, particularly in those patients with unilateral occlusive or dilatative disease; in most cases, however, the distal enhancement is bilaterally adequate for the diagnosis. As far as image degradation from the veins is concerned, previous studies have shown that venous enhancement occurs after approximately 120 s; nevertheless, there might be venous enhancement in cases of cutaneous trophic lesions or in patients with arteriovenous fistulas or varices. In our experience, and in accordance with other studies, venous enhancement did not degrade image quality in any case [7]. A practical contrast medium administration strategy for peripheral CTA is shown in Table 4.

Renal Arteries

When scanning only the renal arteries, the anatomical volume to be covered is obviously shorter than when studying the entire abdominal aorta and peripheral vessels. Therefore the total amount of contrast medium will be targeted to the actual scan time (which of course depends on the CT scanner available). Once the contrast medium arrival time has been determined (either by the bolus test or the trigger technique), even when scanning with a high spatial resolution (4×1, 16×0.75) the scan time will not exceed 15 s. This protocol allows

the use of a limited amount of contrast medium (80 ml at 4 ml/s), yet yields excellent opacification (Fig. 4). A practical contrast medium administration strategy for renal CTA is shown in Table 5.

Three-Dimensional Post-processing for CTA

When performing an MDCT peripheral vascular study, a large amount of data is routinely produced. For easier management, the volume data set is then transmitted to a dedicated workstation where all CTA studies are analyzed using three-dimensional rendering software [4, 5]. The three-dimensional data set analysis uses several types of reconstruction algorithms and should be considered part of the MDCT examination.

Rapid scrolling of the axial image is always carried out as the first step of the reviewing process in all MDCT angiography examinations; the reader can select different planes of examination and can then apply all reconstruction algorithms provided by the workstation: multiplanar reformatting (MPR), maximum intensity projection (MIP), thin MIP, and volume rendering (VR).

The creation of MIP reconstructions usually involves removal of bony structures from the source image, which can be time-consuming, although, in our experience, MIP represents the best algorithm to display very fine details of PAD. VR has the advantage of allowing fairly detailed assessment of the vascular tree without

Table 4. Peripheral CTA: contrast medium injection strategy

Scan Det × mm	Delay (s)	Flow Rate (mL/s)	Volume (mL)	Expected Scan Time (s)
4×3	28	4 to 5	140	35 to 50
8×1.25	TB or Tr + 8	4 to 5	130	32
16×1.25	TB or Tr + 10	4 to 5	110	25 to 28
Data refer to high Iodine concentration solution (370/400 mgI/mL); TB = Test Bolus, Tr = Trigger				

Table 5. Renal CTA: contrast medium injection strategy

Scan Det × mm	Delay (s)	Flow Rate (mL/s)	Volume (mL)	Expected Scan Time (s)
4 × 1	TB or Tr	4 to 5	120	25
8 × 1.25	TB or Tr	4 to 5	90	18
16 × 0.625	TB or Tr	4 to 5	80	15
× 0.75				
× 0.5				
Data refer to high Iodine concentration solution (370/400 mgI/mL); TB = Test Bolus, Tr = Trigger				

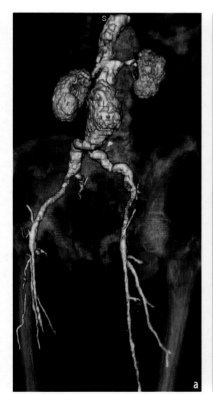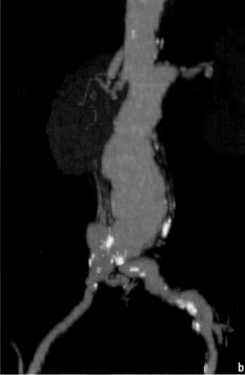

Fig. 5a, b. Patient with AAA and left claudication also presented a severe stenosis of the left renal artery. Both VR (**a**) and MIP (**b**) images clearly show the AAA with atherosclerotic wall changes and calcified plaques, the left renal artery stenosis, and the occlusion of the right SFA

necessarily requiring bony editing (Fig. 5).

Nevertheless, the use of only MIP, thin MIP, and VR may impair the quantification of stenosis, particularly if heavy parietal calcification or endoluminal stents are present (which may even completely obscure the vascular flow). This represents the major drawback of both MIP and VR techniques. The easiest way to assess luminal narrowing and vessel wall disease is to review the transverse source images. Alternatively, longitudinal cross-sections can be obtained using either multiplanar or curved planar reformations (CPR).

CPR provide the most comprehensive cross-sectional display of luminal pathology. Our experience suggests that using either CPR or very thin MIP (reformatted along the vessel course and without bony editing), allows fine anatomical and/or pathological detail of the renal arteries to be achieved. This can be further improved by second-task targeted thinner reconstruction of the kidney area (when a 4×3-mm detector configuration is employed) [8] (Fig. 3).

A recent article by Ota et al. [9] showed that the highest accuracy for stenosis, especially in the pelvic arteries, is achieved by analyzing cross-sectional images rather than simply original axial images. In their study the accuracy rose from 93.5% with original axial images to 99.1% with cross-sectional images, and the difference was even greater in the presence of heavy parietal calcifications, which mainly occur in peripheral occlusive disease at the aorto-iliac segments.

Clinical Applications Overview

Numerous reports have confirmed the robustness of CTA for imaging the aorta and other vessels and its many advantages compared with conventional angiography. In particular, whereas conventional angiography reveals the lumen of an aneurysm, CTA demonstrates the overall aneurysm size and extent, as well as its relationship to adjacent structures (Fig. 6). Van Hoe et al. [10], for example, compared CTA with DSA in 38 patients with abdominal aortic aneurysms; the proximal extent of the 15 juxta- and suprarenal aneurysms was predicted correctly in 14 cases with CTA but in only 12 cases with DSA. There have been additional reports on the utility of helical CTA for imaging suspected traumatic aortic injury [11], for the examination of living renal donors [12], for the staging of malignancy prior to surgery, and for the evaluation of hepatic transplant recipients before and after surgery [13]. For all of these clinical situations, CTA could be combined with additional imaging (e.g., unenhanced, portal venous, delayed).

The use of CTA for imaging the renal arteries was first reported by Rubin et al. [14], although subsequent investigations of CTA for renal artery

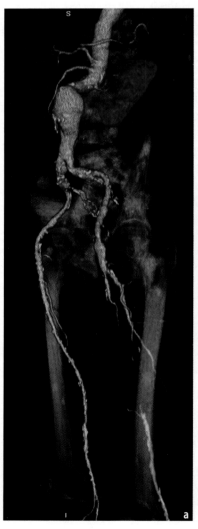
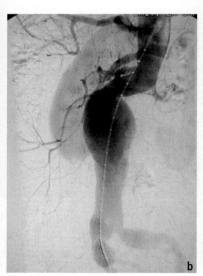
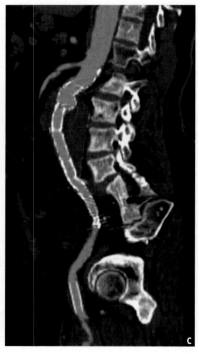

Fig. 6a-c. Patient with AAA. The CTA study with VR technique (**a**) demonstrated an infrarenal AAA, a left common iliac artery stenosis, left common femoral artery dilation, and left SFA occlusion. The patient underwent DSA (**b**) and AAA endovascular repair as well as left common iliac artery stenting, in order to improve the inflow. Post-procedural CTA (**c**) showed complete exclusion of the aneurysmal sac and correct deployment of the iliac stent

stenosis were somewhat disappointing. By the mid to late 1990s, with the use of thinner sections and an optimized technique, reports were published of nearly 100% sensitivity and specificity for the identification of more than 50% renal artery stenoses [16-18]. For the evaluation of patients with suspected renal artery stenosis, CTA is less expensive than magnetic resonance angiography (MRA), can reveal flow within metal stents as well as arterial calcification, and can be used to directly plan for renal arterial angioplasty [18]. However, CTA requires the use of iodinated contrast medium, which is not suitable for patients with renal insufficiency. Multiphasic helical CT, including CTA, was also reported as a replacement for the combination of DSA and intravenous urography for the evaluation of patients being considered as living renal donors. As first reported by Rubin et al. [19], and confirmed by multiple investigations (most recently in patients undergoing laparoscopic renal extraction) [20], there was a very high correlation with findings at surgery for the arterial and venous anatomy. Multiphasic CT permitted the identification of calculi, anatomical variations such as multiple renal arteries, early renal branching, and retroaortic/circumaortic renal veins, and renal masses. Similar techniques can also be used for imaging potential living liver donors, although in this instance MRA is advantageous, because MR cholangiography can easily be performed at the same sitting, permitting anatomical variants that might preclude donation to be identified.

CTA has been demonstrated to be robust and effective by many authors for the infrarenal aorta and peripheral vessels, with very high sensitivity, specificity, and accuracy compared with DSA. With such a large scan volume, MDCT has replaced DSA for imaging of peripheral arterial occlusive disease, leaving DSA for treatment purposes only.

Low-Dose Scanning

With the advent of MDCT, the total number of vascular examinations performed routinely has dramatically increased (to 1,450 studies performed in the recent past at the Cardio-Vascular Imaging Service, Department of Radiological Sciences, University of Rome "La Sapienza"). This poses requirements for a reduction of the X-ray dose delivered to the patient. With regular amperage (130 mA) the effective CTA dose is 13.8 mSv. At 8.8 mSv, there is a risk of up to 0.02% for inducing cancer in the population over 50 years old, which is currently considered the target population for atherosclerotic disease. For this reason new protocols with low dose are necessary. Our experience suggests that the actual dose delivered to the patient can be reduced to 8.2 mSv for 100 mA and to 3.7 mSv for 50 mA, thus obtaining a critical dose reduction of up to 62%.

However, CT scans with low irradiation dose reduce the signal-to-noise (S/N) ratio of the images, with a subsequent decrease in image quality. A possible solution to this problem is the use of contrast agents with a high iodine concentration; this

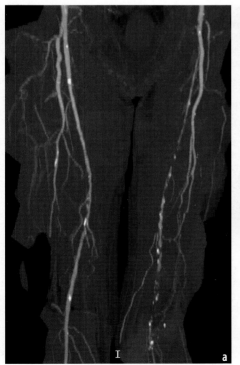
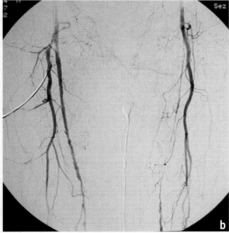

Fig. 7a, b. CTA of the run-off arteries (**a**) performed with a low-dose scan protocol (50 mA) and a high iodine concentration (400 mg I/ml) shows multiple atherosclerotic changes of the right SFA with segmental stenotic lesions and occlusion of the left SFA, as confirmed by DSA (**b**). Lowering the dose delivered to the patient did not affect the diagnostic accuracy, especially with a contrast medium with a high iodine concentration; this should be considered as an alternative CTA scan protocol for slim, young patients

may compensate for the reduction in S/N. Figure 7 shows that diagnostic accuracy is not affected when a contrast medium with a high iodine concentration (400 mg I/ml) is used with low-dose CTA (50 mA).

To be remembered also is that image quality per se is not a critical issue in diagnostic radiology since the ultimate goal is solely the correct diagnosis.

Conclusions

With the continuing advances in MDCT, CTA has continued to evolve. Helical CT and now MDCT have revolutionized non-invasive arterial imaging for an increasing number of examinations, and continue to do so to this day. Conventional angiography will always play a major role in patient care, because interventional vascular procedures require arterial catheterization. However, for diagnostic purposes, CTA, especially when performed on MDCT scanners, has become the imaging modality of choice for many clinical situations, including suspected aortic dissection or transection, aortic aneurysm, suspected pulmonary artery embolism, tumoral staging, and evaluation of potential living renal donors. MRA does compete with CTA, but with the improvements in the spatial resolution of MDCT angiography and the ease of reformation of the imaging volume, the advantages of MRA for some indications have decreased over the past few years. MRA continues to have a primary role when radiation exposure is a concern (especially in young individuals who may need multiple studies over time or when multiphasic imaging is to be performed) or when iodinated contrast is contraindicated (due to renal dysfunction or allergy). The challenges of viewing, interpreting, and storing increasingly large CT data sets have lessened to some extent as picture archiving systems and workstations have kept up with these demands. Multiple types of reformations are now available with a click of a button and within a matter of seconds even volumetric reformations are achievable. However, in our opinion, review of the images in a cine fashion on a CT monitor or workstation remains the mainstay of initial evaluation, even with CTA of the lower extremities. Finally, when interpreting CTA studies, attention must always be paid to the extra-arterial structures, since CT is a global examination, and alternative or additional diagnoses may be present.

References

1. Hu H (1999) Multi slice helical CT: scan and reconstruction. Med Phys 26:5-18
2. Klingenbeck-Regn K, Schaller S, Flohr T et al (1999) Subsecond multislice-computed tomography: basics and applications. Eur J Radiol 31:110-124
3. Rubin GD, Shiau MC, Leung AN et al (2000) Aorta and iliac arteries: single versus multiple detector-row helical CT angiography. Radiology 215:670-676
4. Fishman EK (2000) Real time visualization of volume data: applications in computed tomography angiography. In: Marincek B, Ros PR, Reiser M, Baker ME (eds) Multislice CT: a practical guide. Springer, Berlin Heidelberg New York, pp 125-133
5. Rubin GD, Dake DS, Semba CB (1995) Current status of three dimensional spiral CT scanning for imaging vasculature. Radiol Clin North Am 33:51-70
6. Catalano C, Fraioli F, Laghi A et al (2004) Infrarenal aortic and lower-extremity arterial disease: diagnostic performance of multi-detector row CT angiography. Radiology 231:555-563
7. Rubin GD, Smidt AJ, Logan LJ et al (2001) Multi detector row CT angiography of lower extremity arterial inflow and run-off: initial experience. Radiology 221:146-158
8. Kalender WA, Schmidt B, Zanke M et al (1999) A PC program for estimating organ dose and effective dose values in computed tomography. Eur Radiol 9:555-562
9. Ota H, Takase K, Igarashi K et al (2004) MDCT compared with digital subtraction angiography for assessment of lower extremity arterial occlusive disease: importance of reviewing cross-sectional images. AJR Am J Roentgenol 182:201-209
10. Van Hoe L, Baert AL, Gryspeerdt S et al (1996) Supra- and juxtarenal aneurysms of the abdominal aorta: preoperative assessment with thin-section spiral CT. Radiology 198:443-448
11. Gavant ML, Manke PG, Fabian T et al (1995) Blunt traumatic aortic rupture: detection with helical CT of the chest. Radiology 197:125-133
12. Rubin GD, Alfrey EJ, Dake MD et al (1995) Spiral CT for the assessment of living renal donors. Radiology 195:457-462
13. Nghiem HV, Jeffrey RB Jr (1998) CT angiography of the visceral vasculature. Semin US CT MRI 19:439-446
14. Rubin GD, Dake MD, Napel SA et al (1993) Three-dimensional spiral CT angiography of the abdomen: initial clinical experience. Radiology 186:147-152
15. Galanski M, Propkop M, Chavan A et al (1993) Renal arterial stenoses: spiral CT angiography. Radiology 189:185-192
16. Beregi JP, Djabbari M, Desmoucelle F et al (1997) Popliteal vascular disease: evaluation with spiral CT angiography. Radiology 203:477-483
17. Kaate R, Beek FJ, Lange EE de et al (1997) Renal artery stenosis: detection and quantification with spiral CT angiography versus optimized digital subtraction angiography. Radiology 205:121-127
18. Propkop M (1999) Protocols and future directions in imaging of renal artery stenosis: CT angiography. J Comput Assist Tomogr 23:S101-S110
19. Rubin GD, Dake DS, Semba CB (1995) Current status of three dimensional spiral CT scanning for imaging vasculature. Radiol Clin North Am 33:51-70
20. Kawamoto S, Montgomery RA, Lawler LP et al (2003) Multidetector CT angiography for preoperative evaluation of living laparoscopic kidney donors. AJR Am J Roentgenol 180:1633-1638

III.4

MDCT for Diagnosis of Pulmonary Embolism: Have We Reached Our Goal?

Andreas F. Kopp, Axel Küttner, Stephen Schröder, Martin Heuschmid and Claus D. Claussen

Introduction

Computed tomography (CT) has dramatically changed the diagnostic approach to suspected pulmonary embolism in the last decade. Pulmonary computed tomographic angiography (CTA) is today an accurate test for the detection of pulmonary embolism (PE) and is gaining increased acceptance as a first-line study for diagnosing acute PE (Fig. 1) [1].

In Search of a Gold Standard

Although pulmonary angiography has traditionally been regarded as the gold standard for the diagnosis of PE (Fig. 2), it is undoubtedly a flawed gold standard [2]. In the Prospective Investigation of Pulmonary Embolism Diagnosis (PIOPED) study, the rate of non-diagnostic pulmonary angiography was 3% [3]. Isolated subsegmental pulmonary emboli were seen in 6% of patients, and interobserver variability in the diagnosis of emboli at this level was 66%. There is accumulating evidence illustrating the limitations of this technique for the unequivocal diagnosis of isolated peripheral pulmonary emboli. Two recent analyses of the interobserver agreement rates for the detection of subsegmental emboli with selective pulmonary angiography ranged from only 45% to 66% [4]. Given such limitations, use of this method as an objective and readily reproducible tool for the verification of findings from competing imaging modalities regarding the presence of PE seems questionable, and the status of pulmonary angiography as the standard of reference for diagnosis of PE is in doubt.

The use of nuclear medicine imaging, once the first study in the diagnostic algorithm for PE, is also in decline [5], owing to poor interobserver correlation [6] and the high percentage of indeterminate studies (73% of all studies performed [3]).

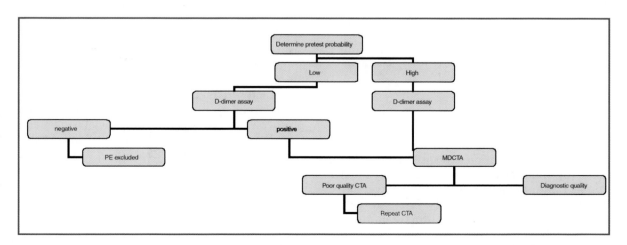

Fig. 1. Clinical algorithm for patients with clinical suspicion of pulmonary embolism (*PE*). *CTA*, computed tomographic angiography; *MDCTA*, multi detector CTA

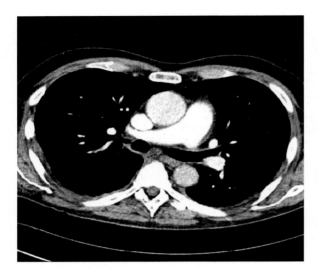

Fig. 2. A 29-year-old male patient with acute chest pain. Pulmonary CTA with low-dose settings was performed to rule out pulmonary embolism. Despite a voltage of only 80 kV and a tube current of 100 mA, the image quality is still diagnostic (collimation 16×0.75 mm, 80 ml Iomeron 400)

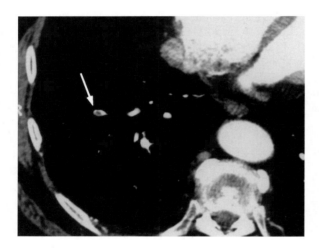

Fig. 3. A 50-year-old male patient with chest pain: transverse contrast-enhanced 16-row multidetector scan with submillimeter collimation (16×0.75 mm, 80 ml Iomeron 400) reveals an isolated subsegmental embolus (*arrow*)

Newer technologies in nuclear medicine, such as single-photon emission CT [7], and revised criteria for the interpretation of ventilation-perfusion scans [8] might help decrease the rate of indeterminate scintigraphic studies. Interobserver agreement for CT is considerably better than that for scintigraphy. Blachere et al. [6] found an interobserver agreement for the diagnosis of PE of 0.72 for CTA and only moderate agreement for ventilation-perfusion lung scanning (0.22).

Furthermore, with the advent of 16-slice multi-detector-row CT (MDCT), traditional technical limitations of CT in the diagnosis of PE appear to have been successfully overcome (Fig. 3) [9, 10]. Therefore, in more recent studies, clinical follow-up with CT has been chosen as the gold standard over pulmonary angiography [4, 11]. It is accepted that PE occurring within 3 months of a CT pulmonary angiogram that showed no signs of PE most likely indicates an initial false-negative examination [12, 13]. This approach may miss small emboli that do not lead to the presentation of symptoms, but such emboli are unlikely to be clinically significant if no evidence of recurrent thromboembolic disease has been noted 3 months or longer after initial presentation [9, 14, 15].

Contrast Medium Injection

The advent of MDCT has necessitated an extensive revision of injection protocols for contrast material (Tables 1 and 2). Faster scanning times allow acquisition during maximal contrast enhancement of pulmonary vessels but pose an increased challenge for the precise timing of the contrast material bolus. Strategies that have the potential to improve the delivery of contrast material for high and consistent vascular enhancement during pulmonary CTA currently include use of high-concentration contrast media (400 mg of iodine/ml, e.g., Iomeron 400) together with automated bolus-triggering techniques [15]. It is essential to achieve a high level of iodine concentration rapidly. This is particularly important using scanners that have a large number of detector rows. A given volume of high-concentration contrast medium will produce higher attenuation in the arteries than the same volume of standard contrast medium (300 mg of iodine/ml). The use of high-concentration contrast medium has the advantages of facilitating post-processing, allowing depiction of smaller vessels and reducing the overall amount of contrast medium required by approximately 30%. Saline chasing has been used for the effective utilization of contrast material and for the reduction of streak artifacts arising from the superior vena cava. Multiphasic injection protocols have proved to be beneficial for general CTA, but so far have not been scientifically evaluated for the diagnosis of PE.

Negative Predictive Value

Patient treatment after a CT pulmonary angiogram that shows no signs of PE is controversial. In a recent study, Kavanagh et al. [16] reported

Table 1. Protocols for suspected acute pulmonary embolism

	4-slice	16-slice scanner
kV/effective mA/rotation time (s)	140/100/0.5	80–120/130/0.5
Detector collimation (mm)	2.5	0.75
Feed/rotation (mm)	15 (ca-cr)	15.0 (ca-cr)
Slice thickness (mm)	3	1.5
Increment	2	1
Kernel	B30f	B30f
IV contrast volume		
(400 mg I/mg)/saline	120/30 ml	80/30 ml
Injection rate		
3 ml/s	3–4 ml/s	
Scan delay (s)	25–30 s (bolus)	25–30 s (bolus)

Table 2. Protocols for pulmonary embolism (*PE*) with a 4-row detector scanner. With four-row technology two separate protocols for evaluation of PE are recommended. A high-speed protocol for dyspneic patients with suspicion of acute PE and a high-resolution protocol with the thinnest collimation, allowing the most detailed display of the pulmonary arteries

	Acute PE	Chronic PE
kV/effective mA/rotation time (s)	120/100/0.5	120/130/0.5
Detector collimation (mm)	2.5	1
Feed/rotation (mm)	15 (ca-cr)	6.0 (ca-cr)
Slice thickness (mm)	3	1.5
Increment	2	1
Kernel	B30f	B30f
IV contrast volume		
(400 mg I/mg)/ saline	120/30 ml	120/30 ml
Injection rate		
3 ml/s	3–4 ml/s	
Scan delay (s)	25–30 s (bolus)	35–50 s (bolus)

a negative predictive value of 99% for MDCT pulmonary angiography for subsequent clinically significant PE. An MDCT pulmonary angiogram with no signs of PE correlates with a low risk of subsequent clinically significant PE.

Outlook

Recently, a new generation of MDCT scanners has been introduced with 64-row technology. Together with shorter gantry rotation, this significantly further increases the volume speed of MDCT. The SIEMENS Sensation 64 scanner with a rotation time of 0.33 s also uses oversampling in the z-direction for better spatial resolution (Fig. 4). This allows isotropic 0.4-mm spatial resolution even at maximum table speed (64×0.6 mm collimation), i.e., the scan of the entire thorax at submillimeter resolution takes less than 5 s. To date, no study has been published for 64-row pulmonary MDCT angiography. However, preliminary results demonstrate that the increased spatial resolution facilitates delineation of even the smallest branches in the periphery of the lung (Fig. 5). Together with the very short scan time due to the better temporal resolution, image quality and robustness of image quality of CTA will be improved. This will also affect the sensitivity and negative predictive value of CTA. In the future, 64-row pulmonary CTA might very well become the new gold standard for the detection of PE.

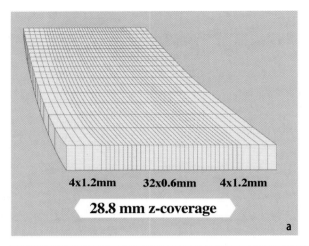

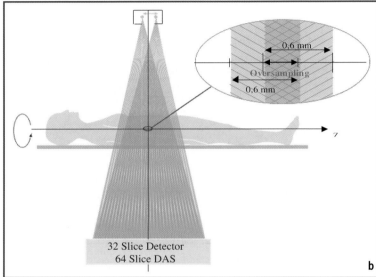

Fig. 4a, b. 64-row technology with 0.4-mm spatial resolution and 0.33-s gantry rotation time (Sensation 64 by SIEMENS Medical). The detector consists of an adaptive array of 32 0.6-mm elements in the center and 4 1.2-mm elements on each side

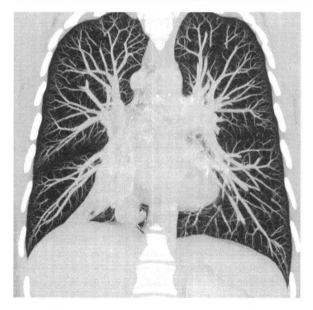

Fig. 5. CTA of the pulmonary vessels using the new 64-row technology demonstrating the 0.4-mm spatial resolution (64×0.6 mm, 60 ml Iomeron 400). The scan of the entire thorax takes less than 5 s

Conclusions

With 16-32-, and 64-row MDCT technology, past limitations of CT for the diagnosis of PE have been effectively overcome. CT is now an attractive means for establishing a safe, highly accurate, and cost-effective diagnosis of PE.

References

1. Ghaye B, Remy J, Remy-Jardin M (2002) Non-traumatic thoracic emergencies: CT diagnosis of acute pulmonary embolism: the first 10 years. Eur Radiol 12:1886-1905
2. Prologo JD, Glauser J (2002) Variable diagnostic approach to suspected pulmonary embolism in the ED of a major academic tertiary care center. Am J Emerg Med 20:5-9
3. The PIOPED Investigators (1990) Value of the ventilation/perfusion scan in acute pulmonary embolism. Results of the prospective investigation of pulmonary embolism diagnosis (PIOPED). JAMA 263:2753-2759
4. Diffin DC, Leyendecker JR, Johnson SP et al (1998) Effect of anatomic distribution of pulmonary emboli on interobserver agreement in the interpretation of pulmonary angiography. AJR Am J Roentgenol 171:1085-1089
5. Schibany N, Fleischmann D, Thallinger C et al (2001) Equipment availability and diagnostic strategies for suspected pulmonary embolism in Austria. Eur Radiol 11:2287-2294
6. Blachere H, Latrabe V, Montaudon M et al (2000) Pulmonary embolism revealed on helical CT angiography: comparison with ventilation-perfusion radionuclide lung scanning. AJR Am J Roentgenol 174:1041-1047
7. Bajc M, Albrechtsson U, Olsson CG et al (2002) Comparison of ventilation/perfusion scintigraphy and helical CT for diagnosis of pulmonary embolism; strategy using clinical data and ancillary findings. Clin Physiol Funct Imaging 22:392-397
8. Stein PD, Gottschalk A (2000) Review of criteria appropriate for a very low probability of pulmonary embolism on ventilation-perfusion lung scans: a position paper. Radiographics 20:99-105
9. Herzog P, Wildberger JE, Niethammer M et al (2003) CT perfusion imaging of the lung in pulmonary embolism. Acad Radiol 10:1132-1146
10. Schoepf UJ, Costello P (2004) CT angiography for diagnosis of pulmonary embolism: state of the art. Radiology 230:329-337
11. Baile EM, King GG, Muller NL et al (2000) Spiral computed tomography is comparable to angiography for the diagnosis of pulmonary embolism. Am J Respir Crit Care Med 161:1010-1015
12. Carson JL, Terrin ML, Duff A et al (1996) Pulmonary embolism and mortality in patients with COPD. Chest 110:1212-1219
13. Goodman LR, Lipchik RJ, Kuzo RS (1997) Acute pulmonary embolism: the role of computed tomographic imaging. J Thorac Imaging 12:83-86
14. Kopp AF, Küttner A, Trabold T et al (2003) Contrast enhanced MDCT of the thorax. Eur Radiol 13:44-49
15. Fleischmann D (2003) Use of high concentration contrast media: principles and rationale–vascular district. Eur J Radiol 45 [Suppl 1]:S88-S93
16. Kavanagh EC, O'Hare A, Hargaden G et al (2004) Risk of pulmonary embolism after negative MDCT pulmonary angiography findings. AJR Am J Roentgenol 182:499-504

SECTION IV

Future Prospects in MDCT Imaging

IV

Introduction

Koenraad Verstraete and Paul M. Parizel

By allowing shorter scan duration, longer scan ranges, and/or thinner sections, multidetector-row computed tomography (MDCT) opens up new horizons, such as interventional MDCT and functional imaging in stroke and oncology. These and other new applications come with the downside of a markedly increased data load and risk for substantially increased radiation dose to the patient. However, a smaller quantity of contrast medium (CM) can be used. In the following section, experts in their fields will address these specific topics related to future applications and advances in MDCT. Interventional MDCT is a safe procedure that offers a wide range of possible minimally invasive interventions with low morbidity and low treatment costs. It will become an alternative and supportive technique to surgery and conventional fluoroscopy [1]. The spectrum of indications before, during, and after interventions includes planning of surgical procedures (e.g., cardiovascular and orthopedic surgery), CT-guided interventions (e.g., puncture, drainage, thermo-ablative procedures, percutaneous vertebroplasty or discectomy, etc.), and post-interventional follow-up (e.g., stent localization and control of transarterial chemoembolization and enteral stents). Special scanning parameters are required to reduce the radiation dose. The field of action of interventional MDCT may increase with the increasing availability of high-precision robotics and smart navigation systems.

The improved temporal resolution of MDCT has opened up new perspectives for *functional imaging*. Contrast-enhanced functional MDCT is a perfusion-based technique. It is also known as perfusion CT imaging. Rapid intravenous bolus injection of a high-concentration iodinated contrast agent is followed by a fast series of images or a volume acquisition. Within each voxel, CT density values change over time and reflect the iodine concentration. The sequential images are combined to generate time-density plots. New-generation MDCT scanners with 16–, 32–, 40–, or 64–detector rows provide excellent temporal resolution. Commercially available software can be used to calculate color-coded functional images (parametric maps) that reflect blood flow (i.e., perfusion, expressed in ml/min per 100 g tissue), blood volume (ml/100 g tissue), and mean transit time of the contrast bolus. With advanced data processing techniques, it is also possible to assess the blood vessel permeability and size of the extracellular compartment within each voxel.

Currently, the major applications of functional MDCT are in stroke, myocardial infarction, and oncology. In *acute stroke*, MDCT provides an excellent way of assessing the functional status of brain tissue. Areas of reversible ischemia demonstrate reduced perfusion, but preserved blood volume. This suggests that auto regulation of the cerebral microcirculation is intact, and hence that the brain tissue is viable. This finding is somewhat comparable to the concept of an ischemic penumbra, which is defined in magnetic resonance imaging as a perfusion-diffusion mismatch. Patients with reversible ischemia are potential candidates for thrombolysis, in order to prevent progression of the ischemic region to a complete stroke. Conversely, when a reduction of both perfusion and blood volume is observed, this indicates irreversible infarction.

In acute *myocardial infarction*, contrast-enhanced MDCT shows perfusion defects as foci of reduced attenuation compared with normal myocardium in the early phase of the bolus (early defect). Residual perfusion defects may persist in the late phase of the bolus. After reperfusion therapy for acute myocardial infarction, evaluation of transmural myocardial microcirculation with functional MDCT can predict wall-motion recovery and help to assess a patient's prognosis. Functional contrast-enhanced MDCT has opened up new perspectives for the assessment of cardiac physiology and the microcirculation.

In *oncology*, contrast-enhanced MDCT is helpful for studying tumor angiogenesis. New blood vessels within a tumor are not only produced in greater number but are also abnormally permeable to circulating molecules, leading to leakage of contrast agents into the interstitial space. Temporal changes in tumor enhancement on MDCT have been shown to correlate with histopathological assessments of angiogenesis. The intravascular phase of contrast enhancement reflects microvessel density; the extravascular phase of enhancement most likely indicates blood vessel permeability. In this way, MDCT provides an insight into the pathophysiology of the tumor. In oncology patients, functional contrast-enhanced MDCT provides important information for tumor diagnosis, treatment selection, and monitoring of therapy.

Another difficult problem with MDCT, the "data explosion," relates to workflow issues, posing questions such as (1) which kind of images should be reconstructed, and at what orientation and thickness should data be reconstructed to provide relevant clinical information, (2) who will perform the post-processing (radiologist or technicians), (3) is three-dimensional visualization a luxury or a necessity, (4) which images are needed, (5) how can we provide the clinicians with relevant images, etc. [2]?

Film is no longer an option and three-dimensional workstations will be used for review of different types of reconstructions (e.g., in different planes or multiplanar reconstruction, maximum intensity projections, shaded surface displays, and volume rendering). The first two are limited to external visualization, while the latter allow for internal or immersive visualization, and can be used for endoscopic-type applications. New imaging and visualization strategies will have to be adapted and optimized to meet the challenge of the increased workload of MDCT.

A final issue covered in the next section deals with adverse events to CM, which occur after the patient has left the radiology department [i.e., renal complications due to contrast-induced nephropathy (CIN) and delayed hypersensitivity reactions].

CIN is still a common cause of hospital-acquired renal failure. Major risk factors include chronic renal insufficiency, diabetes mellitus, conditions associated with decreased effective circulating volume, and use of large doses of CM. Low-osmolar contrast agents have been shown to be less nephrotoxic than ionic, high-osmolar contrast agents. Careful hydration prior to CM administration and use of the lowest dose of CM possible are the best prophylactic measures. Therefore, in MDCT, practical injection strategies will have to be adapted based on physiological and pharmacokinetic principles of enhancement.

Delayed adverse events occur within a time scale of 1 h to 8 days after the administration of an iodinated contrast agent. Skin reactions are usually not serious and seem to be more frequent with non-ionic, isotonic dimers than with non-ionic hypertonic, low-osmolar monomers.

References

1. Vogl TJ, Balzer JO, Mack MG, Herzog C (2003) Interventional MDCT. Eur Radiol 13:M139-M145
2. Prokop M (2003) Multislice CT: technical principles and future trends. Eur Radiol 13:M3-M13

IV.1

Multislice CT: Interventional CT

Thomas J. Vogl and Christopher Herzog

Introduction

Due to a growing demand for minimal invasiveness, computed tomography (CT) is increasingly used as an additional or alternative technique to conventional fluoroscopy or surgery. Its supportive role lies in its use as a reliable diagnostic modality in the pre-interventional work-up and post-interventional follow-up of minimally invasive procedures. Alternatively, it can be used as an interventional technique in its own right. Combining low morbidity, minimal invasiveness, and high cost-effectiveness, in many situations interventional CT is preferable to alternative invasive procedures. With the advent of 16-row multidetector-row (MDCT) technology, the spatial resolution of CT has markedly increased. Currently, volume data sets with an almost isotropic resolution, i.e., a voxel size of ~0.4 mm^3, are feasible. Since high resolution is achieved during one breath hold for stack volumes of up to 1,500 mm^3, pre-therapeutic work-up before musculoskeletal, orthopedic, or cardio surgical interventions is markedly facilitated. Post-interventional CT examinations are a gentle means of follow-up, particularly after vascular interventions such as atherectomy, percutaneous transluminal angioplasty, stenting, port implantation, or bypass or valve surgery. In addition, CT is increasingly used for directly monitoring interventional procedures. Among these procedures are small-needle biopsies, insertion of drainage or gastric tubes, port implantations, post-traumatic fixation of unstable vertebral bodies or the pelvis, cementoplasty/vertebroplasty of osteoporotic/pathological fractures, as well as thermo-ablative procedures for liver, lung, neck, or bone tumors.

In the subsequent sections, the role of MDCT in pre-therapeutic work-up, intra-therapeutic monitoring, and post-therapeutic follow-up is reviewed and critically discussed for several indications. In addition, several useful scan protocols are provided.

Technical Aspects of Interventional MDCT

For CT-guided interventions, two different imaging techniques are useful: sequential CT and continuous CT fluoroscopy. Since the sequential approach usually results in higher effective radiation doses [1] and lower diagnostic accuracy for punctures, spiral CT fluoroscopy is currently regarded as the technique of choice [2]. Depending on the clinical problem, in our department both approaches are applied separately and in combination.

Since the slice thickness can theoretically be decreased to 0.5 mm, sequential scans are particularly useful for interventions on small structures. However, the overall irradiation dose is higher and thus we prefer CT fluoroscopy. In our patients we observed a mean intervention time of 17.9 s (range 1.2–101.5 s), mean milliampere values of 13.2 mA (range 10–51 mA), a mean radiologist irradiation dose per procedure of 0.025 mSv, mean individual procedure doses of 0.0275 mSv (range 0.007–0.048 mSv), and a negligible finger irradiation dose.

Scanning parameters and effective radiation dose measurements generally show large variations, depending on the manufacturer and the CT type. Table 1 provides typical values for currently available Siemens Somatom scanners, i.e., the Somatom Volume Zoom and the Sensation 16.

Spectrum of Indications

MDCT for Planning of Interventional Procedures

Pre-therapeutic indications for MDCT currently comprise planning examinations before interventions. In our clinic, planning CT examinations are

Table 1. Scanning parameters for interventional multidetector-row CT[1]

Sequential Scans[2]:	150 mAs 120 kV 0.5 - 10.0 mm slice thickness single slices
CT-Fluoroscopy[3]:	21 mAs 130 kV 0.8 - 24.0 mm slice thickness single slices
Combi-Mode[4]:	150 mAs 120 kV 16 × 0.8 mm - 1 × 24.0 mm slices up to 16 slices simultaneously

[1] Parameters valid only for the Siemens Somatom Plus 4 VZ and the Sensation 16; [2] Biopsy Mode®; [3] CareVision®; [4] Biopsy Combi®

performed prior to various orthopedic, cardio-surgical, vascular-surgical, and angiographic procedures.

Before complex orthopedic procedures, pre-operative CT scanning may facilitate planning of both the surgical approach and the operative technique. Thus in cases of switch-osteotomy of the femoral shaft or head, the surgeon can determine exactly the cutting angle of the osteotomy by using three-dimensional volume-rendered reformations. The risk of failure or re-operation is consequently minimized (Fig. 1).

In patients scheduled for cardiosurgery, MDCT is predominantly performed prior to total endoscopic coronary bypass grafting. It has been shown that MDCT not only provides valuable information on the degree and localization of coronary artery calcifications, but also rather reliably depicts the cardiac course of the vessels, i.e., is able to bridge the myocardium or epicardiac fatty tissue

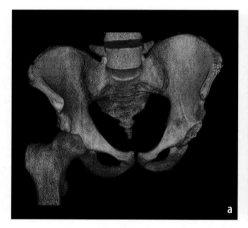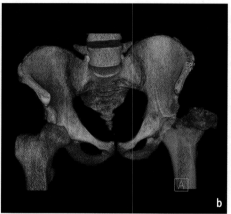

Fig. 1a, b. A 21-year-old woman with known Legg-Calvé-Perthes disease scheduled for a switch osteotomy of the femoral shaft. Preoperative MDCT allowed for perfect simulation of the postoperative outcome and thus made exact planning of the procedure possible

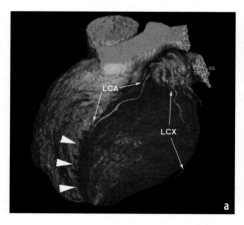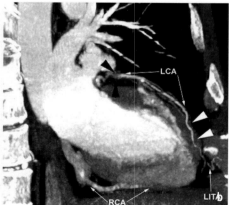

Fig. 2a, b. MDCT findings in a patient scheduled for total endoscopic coronary artery bypass grafting (TECAB). Coronary angiography as well as MDCT revealed a 90% stenosis of the proximal left coronary artery (*LCA*) (segment 6, *black arrowheads*). However, only MDCT showed that the intended site of distal bypass touch-down (segment 7) was hidden deep inside the myocardium (*white arrowheads*). Thus, the surgical approach was altered accordingly and a more-distal site for the distal bypass anastomosis was chosen (left internal thoracic artery, LITA)

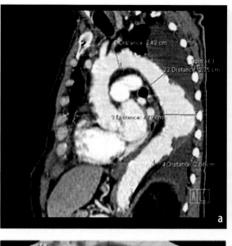
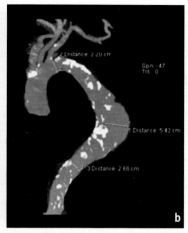

Fig. 3a-d. A 56-year-old patient showing a large sacciform aneurysm of the descending aorta (Stanford type B) before (**a-c**) and after endovascular grafting (**d**). Pre-interventional MDCT is useful to assess the real length of the aneurysm, the minimum and maximum aortic diameter, the diameter of the aneurysm neck, and the diameter of the iliac arteries. In particular, multiplanar reformation (**a**) and three-dimensional volume rendering (**b**) of the CT data sets combined with semi-automatic vessel tracking helps to determine the exact diameters

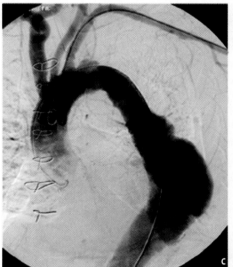
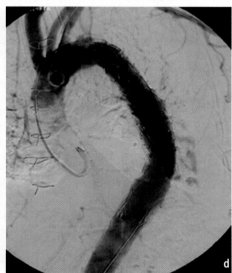

[3]. MDCT is thus able to provide detailed information on the coronary target site and therefore helps the surgeon to choose the most suitable surgical approach (Fig. 2).

Before vascular interventions, MDCT is often performed in patients who need endovascular or open surgical repair of aortic aneurysms and dissections. Multiplanar reformation of CT data sets combined with semi-automatic vessel tracking and measurement tools can very precisely depict the real length of aneurysms, the minimum and maximum aortic diameter, the diameter of the aneurysm neck and, in the case of endovascular stenting, the diameter of the iliac arteries [4-8]. This information helps the surgeon as well as the interventional radiologist to precisely plan the procedure, determine the necessary stent size, and consequently to minimize the duration and risk of the intervention (Fig. 3).

MDCT-Guided Minimally Invasive Interventions

Advances in CT fluoroscopy and adjuvant techniques enable more and more different interventions to be performed. The spectrum of possible indications comprises drainage of abscesses [9, 10] and pneumothoraces [11], punctures of abdominal and thoracic masses and lesions [12-17], percutaneous discectomy of herniated discs, lumbar spine or pelvic interventions [18, 19], percutaneous administration of chemotherapeutic agents [20–22], thermo-ablative procedures [23-25], and percutaneous vertebroplasty [26].

Minimally invasive drainage of abscesses [9, 10], complex pneumothoraces [11], or encapsulated pleural effusions are classic applications for CT. The mortality associated with undrained abdominal abscesses is high, with a rate of between 45% and 100% [9]. The main indications for catheter drainage include treatment or palliation of sepsis associated with an infected fluid collection and alleviation of the symptoms that may be caused by large fluid collections such as pancreatic pseudocele or a lymphocele. In the abdomen single liver abscesses may be drained with ultrasound guidance only [27], whereas multiple liver abscesses or pancreatic abscesses usually require CT guidance [9, 28, 29]. Liver abscesses as well as renal and perirenal abscesses in general are amenable to direct percutaneous drainage. Common percutaneous routes for draining pelvic abscesses include a transgluteal, paracoccygeal-infragluteal, or perineal approach through the greater sciatic foramen [10].

Drainage of simple pneumothoraces or pleural effusions can usually be performed using ultrasound guidance and thus normally does not require the use of CT. However, in cases of complex pneumothoraces or encapsulated pleural effusions, CT guidance may aid access to the regions of interest [27, 28, 30].

Despite improved techniques, the most common complication of percutaneous CT-guided lung biopsy remains the occurrence of a pneumothorax during or after the intervention. The incidence of this complication in the literature ranges between 19% and 60%. Saji et al. [31] studied 289 consecutive patients who underwent biopsy and found that greater lesion depth, wider trajectory angle, and the predicted increased forced vital capacity were independent risk factors for pneumothorax. The lowest rates of pneumothorax were achieved by combining several different puncture techniques [31].

Punctures of musculoskeletal, abdominal, and thoracic masses or lesions may also be performed very accurately using CT guidance [12-17, 32, 33], showing overall diagnostic accuracy ranges between 71% and 92% depending on the localization of the mass/lesion, the technique, and the reporting group.

Hau et al. [17] evaluated the accuracy of CT-guided biopsies of musculoskeletal lesions compared with fine-needle aspiration. In a large series of 359 patients, they found only 63% accuracy for the latter, but 74% for CT-guided biopsies. Pelvic lesions (81%) yielded a higher accuracy than non-pelvic (68%) or spinal lesions (61%). Interestingly, in patients with infectious diseases the accuracy decreased to 50%.

The impact of CT visualization upon the accuracy of punctures of abdominal and thoracic masses has also been examined by Kirchner et al. [1], who found a sensitivity of 71% for CT fluoroscopy compared with 68% for sequential CT. Other groups have achieved 91% accuracy in puncture of thoracic masses by using an unusual trans-sternal approach [16], and 92.6 % with a standard trans-thoracic approach [34]. Similar results were observed by Froelich et al. [35] for fine needle biopsies of the thorax. However, for CT fluoroscopy, reduced procedure times and fewer pleural needle passages were found compared with conventional CT assistance [35].

The irradiation dose is still considered the main limitation to the use of CT interventions [36]. However, Teeuwisse et al. [2] assessed the average effective irradiation doses for 96 CT-guided interventions for sequential CT and continuous CT fluoroscopy and found values of 13.5 mSv and 9.3 mSv for drainages (n=16), 8 mSv and 6.1 mSv for biopsies (n=49), and 2.1 mSv and 0.8 mSv for coagulations of osteoid osteoma (n=31). They concluded that for interventional CT, the effective irradiation doses to the patient were in the same range as those for regular diagnostic CT examinations [2]. Comparable results have been reported by Carlson et al. [37], who observed markedly decreased patient radiation doses and total procedure time for CT fluoroscopy compared with conventional CT guidance. Furthermore, several techniques have been developed to further reduce the irradiation dose and increase the diagnostic accuracy. These include devices such as CT-integrated robots [38], electromagnetic virtual target systems [39], and specific needle holders [40]. A very interesting observation was made by Gianfelice et al. [41], who investigated the effect of the learning process on procedure times and radiation exposure for CT fluoroscopy-guided percutaneous biopsy procedures. Their study shows that after an initial learning period, both the mean procedure and fluoroscopy times are reduced, thereby increasing patient turnover and decreasing radiation exposure to the patient and the operator [41].

In addition to the classic indications, the range of possible interventions has been expanded over the last few years by the introduction of several new procedures such as various lumbar spine interventions, percutaneous pedicle screw insertion in the spine or pelvis [18, 19, 33, 42], percutaneous vertebroplasty [26], thermo-ablative procedures [23-25], percutaneous administration of chemotherapeutic agents [20-22, 43] and several other rather unusual CT-guided procedures [44-46].

Lumbar spine interventions include biopsies of the lumbar vertebrae or intervertebral disk, mainly through a transpedicular or posterolateral approach and the foraminal injection of steroids in patients with radicular symptoms secondary to degenerative change [19]. CT-guided lumbar sympatholysis (LSL) in advanced peripheral arterial occlusive disease is also a very successful procedure. Huttner et al. [47] performed LSL in 138 cases with Fontaine stages III (13%) and IV (87%) and evaluated early and long-term results after 1-5 years. They observed an initial improvement in 79% and a long-term success (>1 year) in 38% of all patients. Although in 49% of cases the dis-

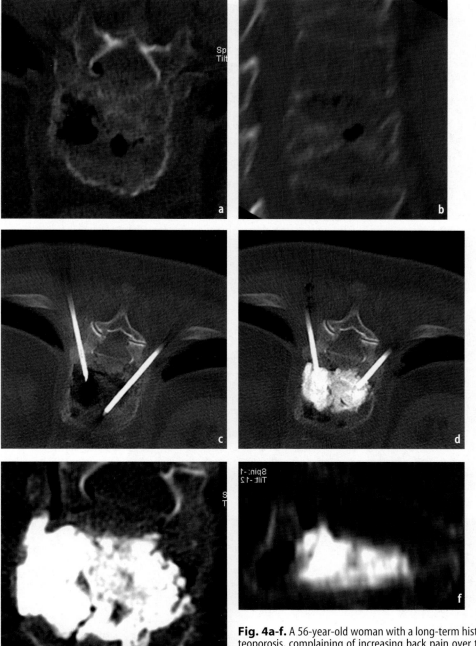

Fig. 4a-f. A 56-year-old woman with a long-term history of postmenopausal osteoporosis, complaining of increasing back pain over the last 4 weeks. MDCT revealed an osteoporotic impression fracture of the ground and deck plate of thoracic vertebra 12 (**a**, **b**). Vertebroplasty was performed via both pedicles using two 12-G needles (**c**, **d**). After instillation of bone cement (Vertebroplastic) a sufficient stabilization of the thoracic vertebra was achieved (**e**, **f**). Pain markedly decreased in the subsequent weeks

ease still progressed, the long-term outcome was significantly better than a control group with conservative treatment only [47]. With the lateral approach for neurolysis in cases of pelvic pain due to advanced cancer, Wilsey et al. [48] recently introduced a very fast but safe approach to the presacral plexus. Another rather new but also promising technique is percutaneous kyphoplasty/vertebroplasty. Both have proved to be safe and effective but are still technically demanding procedures. They can be useful in the treatment of painful osteoporotic vertebral compression fractures that do not respond to conventional treatments [49-54]. Kyphoplasty offers the additional advantage of realigning the spinal column and regaining height of the fractured vertebra. This may help to decrease secondary pulmonary, gastrointestinal, or other morbidity related to these fractures (Fig. 4) [51].

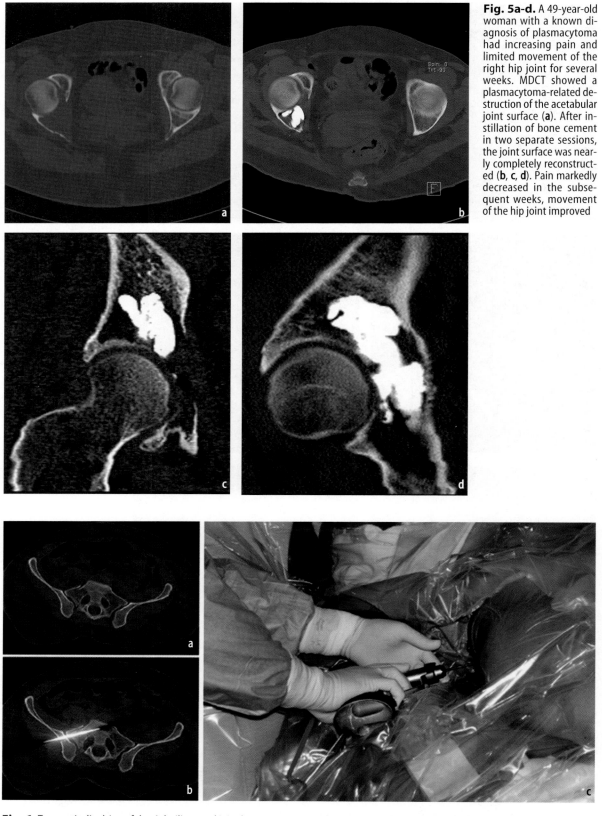

Fig. 5a-d. A 49-year-old woman with a known diagnosis of plasmacytoma had increasing pain and limited movement of the right hip joint for several weeks. MDCT showed a plasmacytoma-related destruction of the acetabular joint surface (**a**). After instillation of bone cement in two separate sessions, the joint surface was nearly completely reconstructed (**b**, **c**, **d**). Pain markedly decreased in the subsequent weeks, movement of the hip joint improved

Fig. 6. Traumatic divulsion of the right ilio-sacral joint by percutaneous screw insertion. Shown are the diagnostic findings before (**a**) and after (**b**) the intervention as well as a peri-interventional photograph (**c**). Although CT guidance requires a significantly higher radiation dose than conventional fluoroscopy computer-assisted surgery, it allows for exact positioning of the screws and thus leads to markedly reduced displacement-related complications

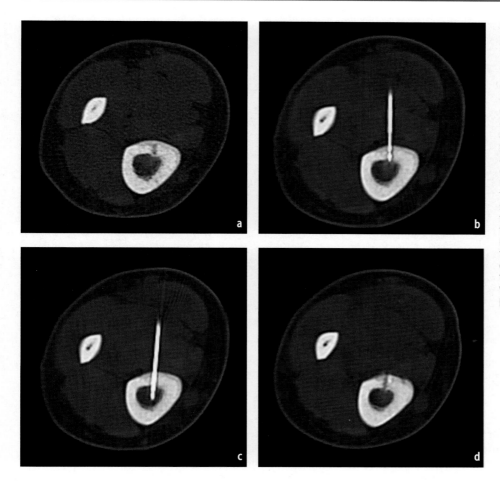

Fig. 7a-d. A 17-year-old patient with severe pain in the upper right calf for 3 months. MRI revealed a 1-mm osteoid osteoma in the upper right tibia. MD-CT shows an intracortical oval lesion with typical central osteolysis (nidus) and reactive thickening of the corticalis (**a**). Findings are most likely due to an osteoid osteoma. CT fluoroscopy was performed in the course of a non-invasive radiofrequency ablation of the lesion (**b, c**). After treatment a local necrosis is observed (**d**). At the time of the follow-up examination 1 month after therapy the patient was completely free of pain

Cementoplasty can be performed not only in patients with (inherent) osteoporotic vertebral compression fractures [49, 50, 53], but also for the effective treatment of extra-vertebral osteolysis [55, 56] or bone metastases (Fig. 5) [57].

Percutaneous pedicle screw insertion in the lumbar or thoracic spine as well as for unstable pelvic fractures is another recently introduced CT-guided intervention (Fig. 6) [18]. Slomczykowski et al. [18] found that standard CT guidance requires a higher radiation dose than conventional fluoroscopic control, but that the CT radiation dose can be significantly decreased by optimization of the scanner settings. They concluded that the advantages of computer-assisted surgery justify CT scans, when based on correctly chosen indications [18].

Thermo-ablative procedures such as radiofrequency (RF) [33, 58] or laser-induced thermotherapy (LITT) [25, 43] have gained much attention during the last few years as alternative treatments for malignant and benign lesions almost anywhere in the body. LITT with MDCT-guided placement of the thermostable catheters allows precise positioning of the needles [25].

In addition to the non-invasive "resection" of liver metastases, RF may also be used as a minimally invasive treatment of osteoid osteomas, showing a satisfactory rate of responsiveness (Fig. 7) [59, 60].

Rather unusual but interesting applications of CT-guided interventions include non-fluoroscopic placement of inferior vena cava filters [44], CT-guided transbronchial biopsies [45], and percutaneous jejunostomy using CT fluoroscopy [46].

MDCT for Follow-Up of Interventional Procedures

MDCT also has an established role in the post-interventional follow-up of surgical/radiological procedures. It may be useful for the control of stent

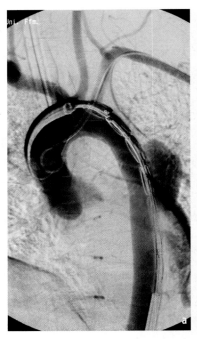 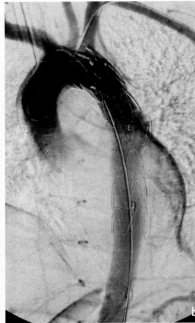 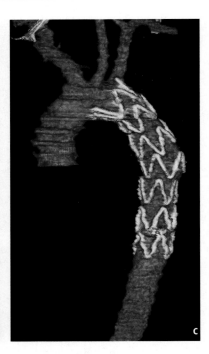

Fig. 8a-c. A 28-year-old man with Marfan syndrome showing a balloon-like aneurysm of the descending aorta. Fluoroscopic stent implantation was performed in cooperation with the Department of Thoracic and Cardiac Surgery. Post-interventional CT control shows the exact placement of the aortic stent distal to the left subclavian artery

localization after aortic stent placement (Fig. 8) [6], for the visualization of the chemotherapeutic agent after transarterial chemoembolization [43, 61], or to control the position of non-covered CHOO enteral stents, placed in the esophagus, stomach, duodenum, and jejunum under conventional fluoroscopy [62].

Conclusions

In conclusion, MDCT has a wide range of indications prior, during, and after minimally invasive interventions. It is a relatively safe procedure that helps to keep treatment costs as well as morbidity low. Although manual puncturing of structures smaller than 8 mm still appears unlikely, the growing availability of high-precision robotics [38, 63] or smart navigation systems may not only help to further increase the accuracy of the puncture but also to reduce the radiation dose of both patient and interventional radiologist. One can expect that in the future, new layer-detector arrays or flat panel technology will further increase diagnostic accuracy and hence widen the spectrum of indications for interventional MDCT. Further information on imaging-guided interventions has been made available on a multi-institutional computer database containing more than 1,000 separate interventions [64]. These data can be used for quality assurance and research purposes.

References

1. Kirchner J, Kickuth R, Laufer U et al (2002) CT fluoroscopy-assisted puncture of thoracic and abdominal masses: a randomized trial. Clin Radiol 57:188-192
2. Teeuwisse WM, Geleijns J, Broerse JJ et al (2001) Patient and staff dose during CT guided biopsy, drainage and coagulation. Br J Radiol 74:720-726
3. Herzog C, Dogan S, Diebold T et al (2003) Multi-detector row CT versus coronary angiography: preoperative evaluation before totally endoscopic coronary artery bypass grafting. Radiology 229:200-208
4. Erbel R, Alfonso F, Boileau C et al (2001) Diagnosis and management of aortic dissection. Eur Heart J 22:1642-1681
5. Czermak BV, Waldenberger P, Fraedrich G et al (2000) Treatment of Stanford type B aortic dissection with stent-grafts: preliminary results. Radiology 217:544-550
6. Balzer JO, Doss M, Thalhammer A et al (2003) Urgent thoracic aortal dissection and aneurysm: treatment with stent-graft implantation in an angiographic suite. Eur Radiol 14:14
7. Kramer S, Gorich J, Aschoff A et al (1998) Diagnostic value of spiral-CT angiography in comparison with digital subtraction angiography before and after peripheral vascular intervention. Angiology 49:599-606
8. Sun Z, Winder R, Kelly B et al (2004) Diagnostic value of CT virtual intravascular endoscopy in aortic stent-grafting. J Endovasc Ther 11:13-25
9. Harisinghani MG, Gervais DA, Hahn PF et al (2002) CT-guided transgluteal drainage of deep pelvic abscesses: indications, technique, procedure-related

complications, and clinical outcome. Radiographics 22:1353-1367

10. Men S, Akhan O, Koroglu M (2002) Percutaneous drainage of abdominal abcess. Eur J Radiol 43:204-218

11. Chang YC, Wang HC, Yang PC (2003) Usefulness of computed tomography-guided transthoracic small-bore coaxial core biopsy in the presence of a pneumothorax. J Thorac Imaging 18:21-26

12. Agid R, Sklair-Levy M, Bloom A et al (2003) CT-guided biopsy with cutting-edge needle for the diagnosis of malignant lymphoma: experience of 267 biopsies. Clin Radiol 58:143-147

13. Liermann D, Kickuth R (2003) CT fluoroscopy-guided abdominal interventions. Abdom Imaging 28:129-134

14. Baldwin DR, Eaton T, Kolbe J et al (2002) Management of solitary pulmonary nodules: how do thoracic computed tomography and guided fine needle biopsy influence clinical decisions? Thorax 57:817-822

15. Gossot D, Girard P, Kerviler E de et al (2001) Thoracoscopy or CT-guided biopsy for residual intrathoracic masses after treatment of lymphoma. Chest 120:289-294

16. Gupta RK, Cheung YK, Al Ansari AG et al (2002) Diagnostic value of image-guided needle aspiration cytology in the assessment of vertebral and intervertebral lesions. Diagn Cytopathol 27:191-196

17. Hau A, Kim I, Kattapuram S et al (2002) Accuracy of CT-guided biopsies in 359 patients with musculoskeletal lesions. Skeletal Radiol 31:349-353

18. Slomczykowski M, Roberto M, Schneeberger P et al (1999) Radiation dose for pedicle screw insertion. Fluoroscopic method versus computer-assisted surgery. Spine 24:975-982; discussion 983

19. Hamze B, Bossard PH, Bousson V et al (2003) Interventional lumbar spine radiology. J Radiol 84:253-262

20. Arrive L, Rosmorduc O, Dahan H et al (2003) Percutaneous acetic acid injection for hepatocellular carcinoma: using CT fluoroscopy to evaluate distribution of acetic acid mixed with an iodinated contrast agent. AJR Am J Roentgenol 180:159-162

21. Engelmann K, Mack MG, Straub R et al (2000) CT-guided percutaneous intratumoral chemotherapy with a novel cisplatin/epinephrine injectable gel for the treatment of inoperable malignant liver tumors. Fortschr Rontgenstr 172:1020-1027

22. Vogl TJ, Engelmann K, Mack MG et al (2002) CT-guided intratumoural administration of cisplatin/epinephrine gel for treatment of malignant liver tumours. Br J Cancer 86:524-529

23. Tacke J (2003) Percutaneous radiofrequency ablation–clinical indications and results. Fortschr Rontgenstr 175:156-168

24. Vogl T, Mack M, Straub R et al (2001) Thermal ablation of liver metastases. Current status and prospects. Radiologe 41:49-55

25. Vogl TJ, Mack M, Straub R et al (2000) Percutaneous interstitial thermotherapy of malignant liver tumors. Fortschr Rontgenstr 172:12-22

26. Peh WC, Gilula LA (2003) Percutaneous vertebroplasty: indications, contraindications, and technique. Br J Radiol 76:69-75

27. Sheafor D, Paulson E, Simmons C et al (1998) Abdominal percutaneous interventional procedures: comparison of CT and US guidance. Radiology 207:705-710

28. Takeuchi Y, Okabe H, Myojo S et al (2002) CT-guided drainage of a mediastinal pancreatic pseudocyst with a transhepatic transdiaphragmatic approach. Hepatogastroenterology 49:271-272

29. Ferrucci J, Mueller P (2003) Interventional approach to pancreatic fluid collections. Radiol Clin North Am 41:1217-1226

30. Inman D, Lambert A, Wilkins D (2000) Multicystic peritoneal inclusion cysts: the use of CT guided drainage for symptom control. Ann R Coll Surg Engl 82:196-197

31. Saji H, Nakamura H, Tsuchida T et al (2002) The incidence and the risk of pneumothorax and chest tube placement after percutaneous CT-guided lung biopsy: the angle of the needle trajectory is a novel predictor. Chest 121:1521-1526

32. Rogalla P, Juran R (2004) CT fluoroscopy [epub ahead of print] Radiologe

33. Thanos L, Mylona S, Kalioras V et al (2004) Percutaneous CT-guided interventional procedures in musculoskeletal system (our experience). Eur J Radiol 50:273-277

34. Charig MJ, Phillips AJ (2000) CT-guided cutting needle biopsy of lung lesions–safety and efficacy of an out-patient service. Clin Radiol 55:964-969

35. Froelich J, Ishaque N, Regn J et al (2002) Guidance of percutaneous pulmonary biopsies with real-time CT fluoroscopy. Eur J Radiol 42:74-79

36. Paulson EK, Sheafor DH, Enterline DS et al (2001) CT fluoroscopy-guided interventional procedures: techniques and radiation dose to radiologists. Radiology 220:161-167

37. Carlson S, Bender C, Classic K et al (2001) Benefits and safety of CT fluoroscopy in interventional radiologic procedures. Radiology 219:515-520

38. Solomon SB, Patriciu A, Bohlman ME et al (2002) Robotically driven interventions: a method of using CT fluoroscopy without radiation exposure to the physician. Radiology 225:277-282

39. Holzknecht N, Helmberger T, Schoepf UJ et al (2001) Evaluation of an electromagnetic virtual target system (CT-guide) for CT-guided interventions. Fortschr Rontgenstr 173:612-618

40. Mack MG, Straub R, Eichler K et al (2001) Needle holder for reducing radiation burden of examiners in CT-assisted puncture. Technical contribution. Radiologe 41:927-929

41. Gianfelice D, Lepanto L, Perreault P et al (2000) Effect of the learning process on procedure times and radiation exposure for CT fluoroscopy-guided percutaneous biopsy procedures. J Vasc Interv Radiol 11:1217-1221

42. Schroder R, Noor J, Pflugmacher R et al (2004) Short-term CT findings after osteosynthesis of fractures of the vertebral spine. Fortschr Rontgenstr 176:694-703

43. Vogl T, Eichler K, Mack M et al (2004) Interstitial photodynamic laser therapy in interventional oncology. Eur Radiol 14:1063-1073

44. Solomon S, Magee C, Acker D et al (1999) Experimental nonfluoroscopic placement of inferior vena cava filters: use of an electromagnetic navigation system with previous CT data. J Vasc Interv Radiol 10:92-95

45. Shinagawa N, Yamazaki K, Onodera Y et al (2004) CT-guided transbronchial biopsy using an ultrathin bronchoscope with virtual bronchoscopic navigation. Chest 125:1138-1143

46. Davies R, Kew J, West G (2001) Percutaneous jejunostomy using CT fluoroscopy. AJR Am J Roentgenol 176:808-810

47. Huttner S, Huttner M, Neher M et al (2002) CT-guided sympathicolysis in peripheral artery disease-indications, patient selection and long-term results. Fortschr Rontgenstr 174:480-484

48. Wilsey C, Ashford N, Dolin S (2002) Presacral neurolytic block for relief of pain from pelvic cancer: description and use of a CT-guided lateral approach. Palliat Med 16:441-444

49. Peh WC, Gelbart MS, Gilula LA et al (2003) Percutaneous vertebroplasty: treatment of painful vertebral compression fractures with intraosseous vacuum phenomena. AJR Am J Roentgenol 180:1411-1417

50. Larsson S (2002) Treatment of osteoporotic fractures. Scand J Surg 91:140-146

51. Garfin SR, Yuan HA, Reiley MA (2001) New technologies in spine: kyphoplasty and vertebroplasty for the treatment of painful osteoporotic compression fractures. Spine 26:1511-1515

52. Einhorn TA (2000) Vertebroplasty: an opportunity to do something really good for patients. Spine 25:1051-1052

53. Cortet B, Cotten A, Boutry N et al (1999) Percutaneous vertebroplasty in the treatment of osteoporotic vertebral compression fractures: an open prospective study. J Rheumatol 26:2222-2228

54. Cotten A, Boutry N, Cortet B et al (1998) Percutaneous vertebroplasty: state of the art. Radiographics 18:311-320; discussion 320-313

55. Bresler F, Roche O, Chary-Valckenaire I et al (1999) Femoral head osteonecrosis: original extra-articular cementoplasty technique. A series of 20 cases. Acta Orthop Belg 65:95-96

56. Cotten A, Duquesnoy B (1995) Percutaneous cementoplasty for malignant osteolysis of the acetabulum. Presse Med 24:1308-1310

57. Marcy PY, Palussiere J, Descamps B et al (2000) Percutaneous cementoplasty for pelvic bone metastasis. Support Care Cancer 8:500-503

58. Yasui K, Kanazawa S, Sano Y et al (2004) Thoracic tumors treated with CT-guided radiofrequency ablation: initial experience. Radiology 231:850-857

59. DeFriend DE, Smith SP, Hughes PM (2003) Percutaneous laser photocoagulation of osteoid osteomas under CT guidance. Clin Radiol 58:222-226

60. Pinto C, Taminiau A, Vanderschueren G et al (2002) Technical considerations in CT-guided radiofrequency thermal ablation of osteoid osteoma: tricks of the trade. AJR Am J Roentgenol 179:1633-1642

61. Vogl TJ, Eichler K, Zangos S et al (2002) Hepatocellular carcinoma: role of imaging diagnostics in detection, intervention and follow-up. Fortschr Rontgenstr 174:1358-1368

62. Dorffner R, Neumann C, Gergely I et al (2002) First experience with a non-covered CHOO enteral stent in the stomach, duodenum, and jejunum. Fortschr Rontgenstr 174:1018-1021

63. Yanof J, Haaga J, Klahr P et al (2001) CT-integrated robot for interventional procedures: preliminary experiment and computer-human interfaces. Comput Aided Surg 6:352-359

64. Mayo-Smith W, Jayaraman M, Han R et al (2003) Multiinstitutional computer database for recording nonvascular imaging-guided interventions. AJR Am J Roentgenol 181:1491-1493

IV.2

Functional CT Imaging in Stroke and Oncology

Kenneth A. Miles

Introduction

Contrast media are widely used in multidetector-row computed tomography (CT) to improve visualisation of the vascular system and renal tract and to increase lesion-to-tissue contrast. Nevertheless, for patients within the first 6 h of acute stroke, the diagnostic and prognostic ability of conventional CT remains poor. Similarly, despite conventional contrast-enhanced techniques, mass lesions on CT may remain hard to characterize as benign or malignant, both at diagnosis and following cancer therapy. Furthermore, visual assessment of tumor enhancement rarely provides useful prognostic information beyond conventional staging. This paper describes how functional CT techniques can maximize the benefits of administering contrast media and so improve the assessment of patients suffering acute stroke or cancer.

Technical Considerations

Quantification for Contrast Enhancement

Table 1 compares the information that can be obtained using contrast media for anatomical and functional purposes. The additional information from functional CT is obtained by quantifying the amount of contrast medium within a given region or volume element (voxel), usually during a time sequence of CT images [1]. Each CT image displays the X-ray attenuation values within each voxel of the anatomical slice studied as an X-ray attenuation map. Following intravenous administration of contrast medium, the iodine component of the contrast medium causes a local increase in the X-ray attenuation that is linearly proportional to the iodine concentration. The amount of attenuation change for a given concentration of contrast medium depends upon a range of factors including the CT system used, the tube voltage (kVp), and the body region examined (e.g., chest or abdomen) and can be ascertained with a simple phantom (Fig. 1). A greater change in attenuation is observed with a lower tube voltage and functional CT protocols may advocate a tube voltage as low as 80 kVp [2].

The concentration of contrast medium at certain time-points following injection can be used to calculate a range of physiological parameters, including cardiac output and glomerular filtration per gram of renal tissue. At tissue level, it is possible to measure blood flow, blood volume, blood vessel permeability and the size of the extracellular compartment within each voxel. Absolute quantification of physiological parameters requires knowledge of contrast enhancement within the vascular system as well as the tissue of interest. However, a simple measurement of peak tissue concentration of contrast medium, when combined with the dose of contrast medium administered per kilogram body weight, can be used to calculate the ratio of tissue perfusion to average whole-body perfusion, also known as the Standardized Perfusion Value

Table 1. Comparison of anatomical and functional applications of contrast media

Anatomical	Functional
Visualise blood vessels	Determine cardiac output
Visualise renal tract	Assess renal function
Improve lesion-to-tissue contrast	Assess physiology of tissue microcirculation, e.g., perfusion, vascular permeability

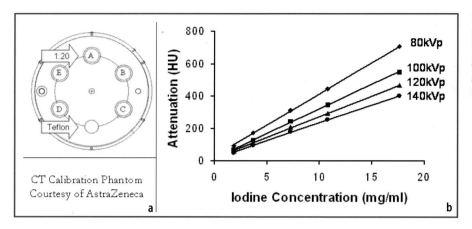

Fig. 1. A calibration phantom containing contrast medium at different concentrations (**a**) can be used to determine the relationship between attenuation and iodine concentration for a range of tube voltages (**b**)

(SPV) [3]. Commercial software is now available to calculate many of these parameters and display them as colour-coded functional images. The derived values are reproducible and have been validated against reference methods [1].

Image Acquisition

Most patients suffering from acute stroke or cancer presently undergo conventional CT, and the simplicity of functional CT means that the necessary images can be readily appended to existing protocols. Functional CT is conceptually similar to CT angiography (CTA) but depicts the circulation at the tissue level rather than visualising discrete vessels. Like conventional angiography, some functional CT protocols require a rapid series of images without table movement following a bolus of contrast medium (Table 2, protocols 1 and 2). Such protocols benefit from allowing determination of multiple physiological parameters within one study, but the volume of tissue examined in the cranio-caudal (Z) axis is restricted by the width of the CT detector tract, i.e., 2 cm on modern mutlislice systems. Other functional CT protocols mimic CTA in that they comprise a spiral acquisition at a set time after injection of contrast medium, the precise time possibly determined using a small test bolus of contrast medium (Table 2, protocol 3). In either case, a rapid injection of high-concentration contrast medium (at least 370 mg/ml) is favored for

Table 2. Example acquisition and processing protocols for functional CT

	1	2	3
Contrast medium			
Concentration	370 mg/ml	370 mg/ml	370 mg/ml
Volume	40 ml	50 ml	50 ml
Injection rate	4–7 ml/s	7–10 ml/s	7–10 ml/s
Slice thickness	2×10 mm	2×10 mm	12 cm spiral
No. images	60	25	1
Image frequency	Every 1 s	Every 2 s	At time of peak enhancement (determined from test bolus)
Tube current	50–100 mAs	100–200 mAs	100–200 mAs
Analysis method	Deconvolution	Compartmental modelling	Compartmental modelling
Parameters calculated	Perf, BV, MTT, vascular permeability	Perf, BV, MTT	Perf normalised to cardiac output
Advantages	Good temporal resolution	Low image noise	Whole-organ imaging
Disadvantages	Image noise Limited anatomical coverage	Reduced temporal resolution Limited anatomical coverage	Perf values only

(*Perf* = perfusion, *BV* = blood volume, *MTT* = mean transit time)

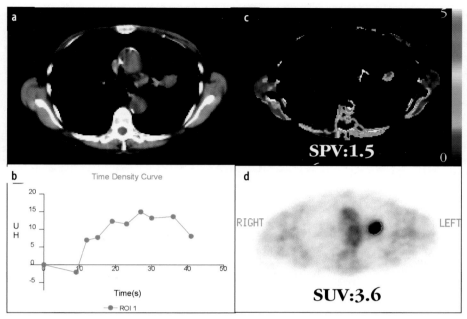

Fig. 2a-d Quantifying contrast enhancement to characterize a left-sided lung nodule and obtain a tumour vascular/metabolic profile. **a** CT prior to contrast enhancement. **b** Time-attenuation curve indicating a peak enhancement of greater than 15 HU at 27 s. **c** Standardised Perfusion Value (*SPV*) image in which the enhancement in each pixel at 27 s has been normalised for patient weight and dose of contrast medium. Enhancement of greater than 15 HU and SPV of greater than 1.5 implies malignancy as does fluorodeoxyglucose (FDG)-PET (**d**). Histology confirmed non-small cell lung cancer. The Standardised Uptake Value (*SUV*) for FDG and SPV indicate a balanced vascular/metabolic profile typical of low-stage lung cancer

two reasons. Firstly, a greater quantity of iodine can be administered in a shorter time, thereby maximizing tissue enhancement and improving signal-to-noise ratios. Secondly, a bolus time of 8 s or less, as required for some analysis methods, can be achieved for a given iodine dose more readily with high-concentration media. Tube current and image frequency are selected with regard to analysis methodology and radiation dosimetry. A higher tube current but lower image frequency may be appropriate when using compartmental analysis as opposed to deconvolution methods (Table 2). A more detailed discussion of analysis methods and protocols can be found elsewhere [1, 4].

Clinical Applications

Acute Stroke

By demonstrating a regional reduction in perfusion and prolongation of transit time, functional CT enables positive diagnosis of acute cerebral ischemia and assessment of prognosis within the first few hours of stroke onset, a time when conventional CT images are typically normal. The size of the ischemic area provides prognostic information and, in the case of embolic stroke, can influence the timing of anticoagulation therapy, as early anticoagulation may be contraindicated unless the infarct is small [5-8]. By comparing perfusion and blood volume images, it is also possible to distinguish reversible from irreversible changes with results that are comparable to diffusion-weighted magnetic resonance imaging [9, 10]. Areas of reversible is-

chemia demonstrate reduced perfusion but preserved blood volume, reflecting preservation of vascular autoregulation and hence tissue viability. Irreversible infarction is characterized by reduced perfusion and blood volume. The term "penumbra" is given to a region of reversible ischemia surrounding an infarct core. Image acquisition without table movement is used to identify reversible ischemia because of the need to compare two physiological parameters. The demonstration of reversible ischemia has been proposed as a means to select patients for thrombolysis, but requires further validation through randomized controlled trials [11].

Oncology

Contrast enhancement in tumors correlates with histological assessments of microvessel density and therefore can be used as an in vivo marker of tumor angiogenesis [12, 13]. Measuring peak enhancement within lung nodules can characterize lesions that are indeterminate on conventional CT; this is increasingly used for assessment of nodules identified by CT screening protocols [14, 15] (Fig. 2). Occult hepatic metastases and other tumor sites undetected by conventional CT may be revealed on functional CT images. By quantifying contrast enhancement within the liver, it is possible to identify patients at risk of subsequently developing overt metastasis and to predict survival [16-18]. CT perfusion measurements can also estimate tumor grade in cerebral glioma and lymphoma [1]. Functional CT can demonstrate the effect of cancer treatment on tumor vascularity and may show a response to drugs that target tumor vessels before any change in tumour size or fluorodeoxyglucose (FDG) uptake is detectable [19]. Measuring a range of physiological parameters within a tumor and assessing vascular heterogeneity produces a profile of tumor vascularity. When combined with measurements of FDG uptake, for example, during PET/CT, a vascular/metabolic profile can be obtained. Such tumor profiles have the potential to classify tumors in a new way. For example, early studies have shown that low contrast enhancement with high FDG uptake is found more commonly amongst high-stage lung cancers and may represent an aggressive tumor type [20].

Conclusions

By exploiting the ability of CT systems to quantify contrast enhancement, functional CT extends the utility of contrast media to include assessment of cardiovascular physiology. Just as Harvey's discovery of the circulation in the seventeenth century significantly advanced medical understanding, so too can functional CT assessments of vascular physiology in ischemic tissue and tumors improve the diagnosis and assessment of patients with stroke or cancer. The variability of clinical course amongst stroke patients with similar clinical presentation, and amongst cancer patients with the same tumor stage, has led to a concept of personalised cancer care in which the patient's treatment is tailored to individual characteristics of their disease. Functional CT can potentially contribute to the delivery of personalised medicine for stroke patients by identifying reversible ischemia amenable to thrombolytic therapy, and for cancer patients by generating vascular profiles that predict tumor aggression, metastatic potential, likely response to radiotherapy, and delivery of chemotherapeutic agents.

References

1. Miles KA, Griffiths MR (2003) Perfusion CT: a worthwhile enhancement? Br J Radiol 76:220-231
2. Wintermark M, Maeder P, Verdun FR et al (2000) Using 80 kVp versus 120 kVp in perfusion CT measurement of regional cerebral blood flow. Am J Neuroradiol 21:1881-1884
3. Miles KA, Griffiths MR, Fuentes MA (2001) Standardized perfusion value: universal CT contrast enhancement scale that correlates with FDG PET in lung nodules. Radiology 220:548-553
4. Miles KA (2003) Perfusion CT for the assessment of tumour vascularity: which protocol? Br J Radiol 76:S36-42
5. Keith C, Griffiths M, Petersen B et al (2002) Computed tomography perfusion imaging in acute stroke. Australas Radiol 46:221-230
6. Wintermark M, Reichhart M, Thiran JP et al (2002) Prognostic accuracy of cerebral blood flow measurement by perfusion computed tomography, at the time of emergency room admission, in acute stroke patients. Ann Neurol 51:417-432
7. Mayer TE, Hamann GF, Baranczyk J et al (2000) Dynamic CT perfusion imaging of acute stroke. Am J Neuroradiol 21:1441-1449
8. Klotz E, König M (1999) Perfusion measurements of the brain: using dynamic CT for the quantitative assessment of cerebral ischemia in acute stroke. Eur J Radiol 30:170-184
9. Wintermark M, Reichhart M, Cuisenaire O et al (2002) Comparison of admission perfusion computed tomography and qualitative diffusion- and perfusion-weighted magnetic resonance imaging in acute stroke patients. Stroke 33:2025-2031
10. Eastwood JD, Lev MH, Wintermark M et al (2003) Correlation of early dynamic CT perfusion imaging with whole-brain MR diffusion and perfusion imaging in acute hemispheric stroke. Am J Neuroradiol 24:1869-1875
11. Latchaw RE, Yonas H, Hunter GJ et al (2003) Council on Cardiovascular Radiology of the American Heart Association Guidelines and recommendations for perfusion imaging in cerebral ischaemia: a scientific statement for healthcare professionals by the writing group on perfusion imaging, from the Council on Cardiovascular Radiology of the American Heart Association. Stroke 34:1084-1104
12. Tateishi U, Nishihara H, Watanabe S et al (2001) Tumor angiogenesis and dynamic CT in lung adenocarcinoma: radiologic-pathologic correlation. J Comput Assist Tomogr 25:23-27
13. Jinzaki M, Tanimoto A, Mukai M et al (2000) Double-phase helical CT of small renal parenchymal neoplasms: correlation with pathologic findings and tumor angiogenesis. J Comput Assist Tomogr 24:835-842
14. Swensen SJ, Viggiano RW, Midthun DE et al (2000) Lung nodule enhancement at CT: multicenter study. Radiology 214:73-80
15. Pastorino U, Bellomi M, Landoni C et al (2003) Early lung-cancer detection with spiral CT and positron emission tomography in heavy smokers: 2-year results. Lancet 362:593-597
16. Platt JF, Francis IR, Ellis JH et al (1997) Liver metastases: early detection based on abnormal contrast material enhancement at dual-phase helical CT. Radiology 205:49-53
17. Dugdale PE, Miles KA (1999) Hepatic metastases: the value of quantitative assessment of contrast enhancement on computed tomography. Eur J Radiol 30:206-213
18. Miles KA, Colyvas K, Griffiths MR et al (2004) Colon cancer: risk stratification using perfusion CT. Eur Radiol 14 [Supp 2]:129
19. Willett CG, Boucher Y, Tomaso E di et al (2004) Direct evidence that the VEGF-specific antibody bevacizumab has antivascular effects in human rectal cancer. Nat Med 10:145-147
20. Miles KA, Griffiths MR, Keith CJ (2004) Preliminary investigations into lung tumour flow: metabolism relationships using perfusion CT and FDG-PET. Nucl Med Commun 25:407

IV.3

MDCT and Data Explosion: Current Technologies and Directions for Future Development in Managing the Information Overload

Geoffrey D. Rubin

Introduction

A great challenge of multidetector-row computed tomography (MDCT) is dealing with "data explosion". A single day's work in a busy clinic may consist of 30 studies, each requiring several hundred images. For carotid and intracranial CT angiograms, we routinely review 375 images (300-mm coverage, reconstructed every 0.8 mm); for aortic studies, we have 450–500 images (~600-mm coverage, reconstructed every 1.3 mm); and for a study of inflow and run-off of the lower extremity, we may generate 900–2,000 transverse reconstructions. One full-body CT examination generates as much as 720 MB of data (scanning a 180-cm person at 1-mm increments produces 1,828 axial images, each 512×512 pixels at 12 bit). Clearly, strategies for efficiently managing this information are necessary. Attempting to manage the information overload by reconstructing fewer images from the data is not a solution, as experience with single-detector CT scanners indicates that longitudinal resolution and disease detection are improved when cross-sections overlap by at least 50% [1].

Therefore, to optimize our clinical protocols and take full advantage of the latest CT technologies, we need to change the way that we interpret, transfer, and store CT data. Film is no longer a viable option: workstation-based review of transverse reconstructions is a necessity. However, the workstations must be improved to provide efficient access to these data, and we must have a way of providing clinicians with images that can be transported to clinics and to the operating room. Alternative visualization and analysis using volumetric tools, including three-dimensional (3D) visualization, must evolve from being considered a luxury to a necessity. We cannot rest on historical precedent to interpret these near-isotropically sampled volumetric data using transverse reconstructions alone [2]. Although the tools for volu-

metric analysis on 3D workstations have evolved over recent years, they have not yet evolved to a level that routine interpretation can be performed as efficiently and accurately as transverse section review.

Both hardware and software developments must occur. While current workstations and visualization software are certainly adequate for volumetrically assessing these MDCT data, the process is time-consuming. In this chapter, I describe current workstation capabilities and briefly discuss areas that require further development for the complete integration of volumetric analysis into the process of interpreting CT data.

Visualization Techniques

Four main visualization techniques are currently in use on clinical 3D workstations: multiplanar reformation (MPR), maximum intensity projection (MIP), shaded surface display (SSD), and volume rendering (VR). The first two techniques are limited to external visualization, while the latter two allow for "immersive" or internal visualization and can be used for endoscopic-type applications.

Multiplanar Reformation

MPR, a convenient and widely available technique for displaying CT data, generates a tomogram corresponding to a slice of 1-voxel thickness. One substantial limitation of traditional MPR is that the visualized structures must lie in one plane. Because it is rare that all structures for which 3D visualization is desired lie within a single plane, MPR is limited in demonstrating the entirety of the anatomical section under study. As structures course in and out of the visualization plane, we may have the false impression of vessel occlusion

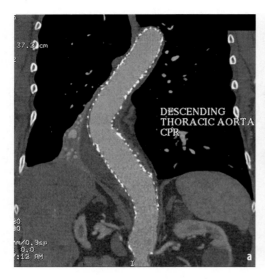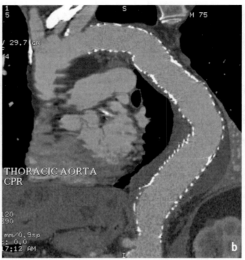

Fig. 1a, b. Curved planar reformations display longitudinal cross-sections of the descending thoracic aorta despite a tortuous course. The lumen of the aorta through the metallic stent graft and thrombus within a descending aortic aneurysm are visible. **a** Curved coronal reformation. **b** Curved sagittal reformation

or stenoses. The solution to this problem is to use curved planar reformations (CPR).

Similar to MPR, CPR generates a single-voxel-thick tomogram, but it is capable of demonstrating an uninterrupted longitudinal cross-section because the display plane curves along the structures of interest. With CPR, the visualization plane typically is created from points that are manually positioned over the structures of interest, as viewed on transverse sections or using MPR, MIP, SSD, or VR visualization techniques. The points are connected to form a curved surface that is then extruded through the volume perpendicular to the desired view to create the CPR. Recently, automated CPR algorithms have been introduced on some clinical workstations to obviate the need for manual identification of centerline points. An important limitation of CPR is that it is highly dependent on the accuracy of the curve. Inaccurately positioned points or insufficient numbers of points can result in the curve "slipping-off" the structure of interest, creating pseudostenoses. Furthermore, a single curve cannot adequately display eccentric lesions; therefore, two curves orthogonal to each other should always be created to provide a more complete depiction of eccentric lesions, particularly stenoses.

CPR is useful for displaying the interior of tubular structures such as blood vessels, airways, and bowel. It is also useful for visualizing structures immediately adjacent to these lumina, such as mural thrombus and extrinsic or exophytic neoplasia, without requiring the data to be edited (Fig. 1).

Maximum Intensity Projection

With this technique, a MIP image is created when a specific projection (e.g., anteroposterior) is selected and then rays are cast perpendicular to the view through the volume, with the maximum value encountered by each ray recorded on a 2D image [3, 4]. As a result, the entire volume is "collapsed" and only the brightest structures are visible (Fig. 2). Variations of this approach include the minimum intensity projection (MinIP), useful for visualizing airways [5], and the raysum or average projection [3], which sums all pixel values encountered by each ray to provide an image similar to a radiograph.

An advantage of MIP over MPR is that structures that do not lie in a single plane are visible in their entirety. A limitation of MIP, however, is that bones or other structures that are more attenuative than contrast-enhanced blood vessels, for example, will obscure the blood vessels. Similarly, when creating MinIP images, air external to the patient obscures the airways and surrounding lung. Two approaches to address the limitations of obscuration are slab-MIP and prerendering editing:

- Slab-MIP images are created when a plane through the data is defined and then "thickened" perpendicular to the plane [6]. The process with which the plane is thickened can be MIP, MinIP, raysum, or VR. By selecting a slab orientation that does not result in overlap of structures with extremely high attenuation (e.g., bones, metal) on structures of interest

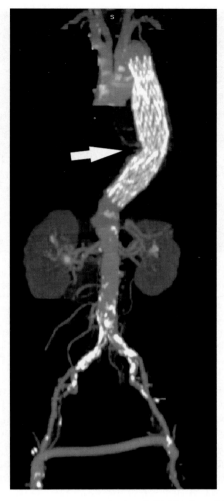

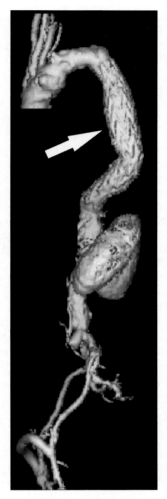

Fig. 2. Maximum intensity projection (MIP). This frontal MIP displays the entirety of the thoracoabdominal aorta and iliac arteries. The metallic portion of a descending thoracic aortic stent graft is shown (*arrow*). The metallic cage obscures the aortic lumen, but is easily visualized because of its attenuation differences compared to the contrast medium-enhanced arterial lumen. Similarly, calcium in the distal aorta and common iliac arteries is easy to identify relative to the enhanced lumen

Fig. 3. Shaded surface display (SSD). Lateral SSD provides greater appreciation of 3D relationships compared to MIP in Fig. 2, but the stent-graft (*arrow*) and arterial calcium deposits are difficult to discriminate from the arterial lumen

(e.g. blood vessels), the latter can be clearly visualized without the need for time-consuming and operator-dependent editing. This approach, however, is generally limited to imaging through slabs that are 5-30 mm thick.

- If an MIP image of a larger subvolume of the data is desired, then the data must first be edited to remove obscuring structures ("prerendering editing"). Techniques for editing CT data are discussed in the subsequent section.

Even after the issues of obscuration have been addressed, some limitations of the MIP technique remain. MIP does not permit the appreciation of depth relationships and, in regions of complex anatomy such as at the neck of an aortic aneurysm, it can be difficult to be confident when the true origin of a branch is visualized versus a foreshortened branch due to overlap of its proximal extent with the aorta itself.

Shaded Surface Display

The shaded surface display (SSD) technique provides exquisite 3D representations of anatomy (Fig. 3), relying on gray scale to encode surface reflections from an imaginary source of illumination [7, 8]. The majority of SSD images created on clinical workstations display a single surface that is the interface between user-selected thresholds. As a result, the 12-bit CT data are reduced to binary data, with each pixel being either within or outside of the threshold range. Some workstations allow several threshold ranges to be defined and displayed with different colored surfaces. In this setting, different tissue types or structures are coded with different colors to facilitate their visualization relative to adjacent structures. For each classification, data segmentation is required, typically by both thresholding and editing, which increases the required processing time arithmetically. Regardless of the number of tissue groups or classes assigned, the selection of the threshold range that defines each class is typically arbitrary and can substantially limit the accuracy of data interpretation, particularly when attempting to grade stenoses. This is particularly true when calcified plaque accompanies regions of arterial stenosis. The plaque typically falls within the same threshold range as blood vessel lumen, resulting in the spurious appearance of a local dilation, rather than a stenosis [9].

Volume Rendering

The final and most complex rendering technique is volume rendering (VR) [10-14]. There are many different versions and interfaces for VR, but the general approach is that all voxel values are assigned an opacity level that varies from total transparency to total opacity (Fig. 4). This opacity function can be applied to the histogram of voxel values as a whole or to regions of the histogram that are classified as specific tissue types [15, 16]. Peaks and plateaus of high, low, or intermediate opacity usually characterize the transfer function. "Walls" slope from the opacity peak or plateau to a baseline of complete transparency in an attempt to account for partial volume effects at the edges of structures. Regions where the opacity curve has a steep slope are referred to as transition zones and are analogous to threshold levels with SSD.

Lighting effects may be simulated in a fashion similar to that for SSD. Because there is no surface definition with VR, lighting effects are applied based upon the spatial gradient (i.e., variability of attenuation within a local neighborhood of voxels). Near the edges of structures, the spatial variation in attenuation changes more rapidly (a high gradient) than in the center of structures (a low gradient). Lighting effects are most pronounced in regions of high spatial gradients. Because lighting effects and variations in transparency are simultaneously displayed, it is frequently useful to view

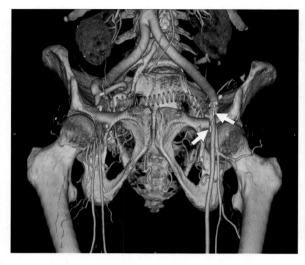

Fig. 4. Volume rendering (VR). Caudally angulated anterior VR of the pelvis from a patient with a patent aortobifemoral bypass graft and an occluded femoral to femoral bypass graft. Three dimensionality is conveyed similar to an SSD, but attenuation differences are visualized based upon the color scale, where metal clips are easily discriminated from the lower attenuation and redder arterial luminal enhancement (*white arrows*)

VR images in color. The color is applied to the attenuation histogram to allow differentiation of pixel values and to avoid ambiguity with lighting effects, which are encoded in gray scale. Other variables such as specular reflectivity, which models the "shininess" of a surface, are available but should be used with caution to avoid confounding the visualization.

Editing CT Data

The challenge of performing efficient and accurate 3D visualization of clinical CT data is to balance the use of visualization techniques that require editing versus those that do not. In general it is preferable to avoid time-consuming editing, but it is occasionally necessary to optimally visualize complex structures. Editing can span from quick and simple interactive cut-plane selection to meticulous 2D region of interest (ROI) selection with intermediate steps being provided by 3D ROI editing, region growing (or connectivity), and slab editing.

Cut-Plane Selection

When viewing SSD and VR images, the use of cut planes is helpful to remove obscuring structures that lie between our viewpoint and the anatomy of interest. Cut planes can usually be oriented arbitrarily but, for the same reasons that MPR images are limited for visualizing curved structures, cut planes are limited for removing curved structures.

3D ROI Editing

This approach to editing is performed when a ROI is selected by drawing a rectangle or more complex shape and extruding this shape through the volume along an appropriate linear path. The selected region is either removed or exclusively retained for rendering. This is a quick technique that requires the drawing of a single ROI that can then be applied to many cross-sections. It is useful for eliminating the air around the chest when creating a MinIP or for removing the spine from data sets containing only the cervical or lumbar regions of the spine.

Unfortunately, 3D ROI editing is not sufficient for removing the pelvis, skull, or large portions of the rib cage, particularly near the thoracic inlet, where a cleavage plane between anatomy of interest and obscuring structures cannot be identified. There are two main approaches for dealing with this problem: region growing (connectivity) and slab editing. Both can be effective but, in general, region growing is more flexible and efficient when combined with Boolean operations such as subtraction.

Region Growing

Region growing (connectivity) is a threshold-based process, where a seed point is selected in the structure of interest and allowed to "grow" into contiguous pixels that are within a defined threshold range. Region growing is rarely adequate as the sole editing tool, because often there are regions of "leakage" where the seed may grow into undesirable structures. To combat this problem, limited cut planes or "scalpel cuts" can be applied over a variable number of sections to disconnect the structures.

A typical application of this technique is the disconnection of the superior gluteal arteries from the sacrum as they exit the pelvis. These predictable sites of leakage between the arteries and bones can be disconnected in seconds. A quick search of the remainder of the cross-sections may reveal problematic osteophytes contacting the aorta, which must be similarly disconnected; then the region growing technique is applied and the aorta and its branches are selected.

There are two approaches to using region growing for editing CT data:
- The first and most intuitive use of region growing is selection of the structure of interest and deletion of all unselected pixels from the data.

This approach has two main limitations. First, the structure of interest may not be identifiable with a single region growing step, as when both sides of an occluded blood vessel are reconstituted distally by collateral flow or a highly stenotic vessel becomes discontinuous with thresholding. Second, the edges of structures will be arbitrarily truncated at the threshold selected for the region growing. Therefore, the edge pixels between the structure of interest and the background are excluded. While SSD images look fine with this approach, MIP images appear as though they have been cut from the data with scissors. This second limitation can be combated with a simple dilation step, where the editing is allowed to "relax" by 1–4 pixels to include these edges. The first limitation, however, cannot be addressed by dilation and thus there is a preferred approach to using region growing, as follows.

- The preferred approach is to use region growing to identify the bones, dilate them by 3–4 pixels to include the edges and subtract them from the original data. A MIP image of 200 transverse abdomen and pelvis sections can be edited in less than 5 min using this approach to display the aortoiliac system free of overlapping bones. The edited data can also be used to create SSD or VR images free of bones, providing a posterior view of the aorta and its branches.

Slab Editing

Slab editing is also an efficient means of editing CT data. Slab editors work by allowing the user to preselect slabs of data of varying thickness. The slabs are displayed as slab-MIP images and a ROI is drawn on each slab. Fewer slabs require less ROI drawing, but more slabs may be required to remove complex structures. For many applications, 5–10 transverse sections are used per slab, improving the efficiency over 2D ROI editing by a factor of 5–10. This technique can be limited in regions such as the pelvis (where the iliac arteries lie close to the pelvic sidewall and the pelvis has a sloping contour) and the skull base adjacent to the circle of Willis.

Section-by-Section 2D ROI Editing

The most time-consuming editing technique is section-by-section 2D ROI editing, where a ROI is drawn individually on each cross-section. This provides the most control, but is extremely time-consuming and should be reserved only for situations where none of the previously described approaches suffices.

Endoluminal Visualization

The ability of helical CT to image the inner surfaces of tubular lumina has led to proposed clinical applications of "virtual endoscopy" to examine the bowel [14, 17, 18], airways [14, 19-21], blood vessels [14], and urinary tract [22, 23]. While the utility of these techniques in the clinical setting has not been fully validated, virtual endoscopy has generated considerable interest among radiologists and other clinicians. While the term virtual endoscopy is catchy, it is vague and is loosely applied to any technique that displays the interior of tubular lumina.

The interior surface of tubular lumina can be visualized with SSD and VR. The basic approach is to identify threshold levels for SSD that exclude pixels of similar attenuation to the lumen (e.g., from -900 to -1,000 HU for air-filled lumina, and in the range of 150-400 HU for contrast-enhanced blood vessels) or to choose an opacity curve for VR that results in complete transparency of the lumen. It is important to recognize that these renderings depict the interface between luminal contrast and extraluminal attenuation, and do not actually show the mucosal or intimal surface. Once the intraluminal pixels have been eliminated or rendered transparent, a view is created to allow unobstructed intraluminal visualization. Toward that end, two main strategies can be employed: orthographic external rendering with cut planes and immersive perspective rendering.

Orthographic External Rendering

Orthographic rendering is the most common type of rendering, particularly for external visualization, and is based upon the assumption that light rays reaching our eyes are parallel, as if structures were viewed with a high-powered telescope from far away. As a result, the proximity of structures to the viewpoint does not influence the size with which they are rendered. Although orthographic rendering is exclusively used for visualization from a viewpoint that is external to the data, it can be used for internal visualization when combined with cut planes that are positioned within the lumen of the structure of interest. This is analogous to cutting a window into a piece of pipe to visualize its interior. This technique is mostly useful for providing regional snapshots but currently cannot provide a continuous display of all interior surfaces within a tubular lumen. Greater inner surface visualization is available with immersive perspective rendering.

Immersive Perspective Rendering

Immersive rendering implies that the viewpoint is within the data set. In order to understand depth relationships from close range, structures should be viewed with perspective. This mode demonstrates spatial relationships similar to the human visual system, where light rays are focused to converge on the retina. The phenomenon of perspective helps us recognize the distance of structures based upon their size, as a structure close to the eye appears larger than a structure further away. The extent to which this effect is observed is determined by the field of view (FOV) of our "virtual lens," which is typically defined as the size of the angle at the apex of a cone of visualization emanating from our viewpoint. A larger angle indicates greater perspective and thus greater disparity in size-distance relationships. Most perspective renderings of CT data are created with a 20°-90° FOV. Both SSD and VR images can be rendered with perspective, and used to create endoluminal views that mimic fiberoptic endoscopy without the mechanical limitations of access to the lumen and view direction.

The greatest challenge of immersive visualization is navigation. "Flying" a virtual endoscope is akin to flying a helicopter. There are three spatial degrees of freedom for position and three spatial degrees of freedom for view direction. When considered with the challenge of appropriate threshold (SSD) or opacity table (VR) selection and color, the complexity of creating these visualizations can be daunting. Furthermore, without some external indication of the view position, either on a 3D model or with MPR, it is easy to lose track of one's location within the lumen. Techniques that automatically create a flight path through the center of a lumen are being developed and are showing promising results. There are likely to be many variations on the performance of virtual endoscopy, aimed at improving efficiency and ease, which will be developed in the near future. However, until these techniques are validated against an established standard, CT endoscopy will remain predominately a research tool.

Systems for CT Data Analysis

There are currently five systems for data analysis available in clinical practice. These systems are not mutually exclusive and may in fact be complementary.

- *Film-based interpretation.* I include this for completeness. In the era of MDCT, film is obsolete for image interpretation, but can be a useful means of transferring partial image sets to referring clinicians.

- *Conventional PACS workstations.* A full discussion of the picture archiving and communication system (PACS) is beyond the scope of this chapter. For MDCT interpretation, PACS offers soft-copy interpretation on workstations that provide easy access to current and prior studies. PACS makes it possible to perform cine-paging of image stacks, dynamically tune window and level settings, make digital measurements, and assess CT attenuation in ROIs; these are invaluable daily tools that film does not offer. However, most PACS stations do not provide tools for 3D visualization.

- *3D and MPR on the CT scanner.* In some low-volume practices, creating alternative visualizations on the CT console may be a practical solution. In a busy practice, routinely using the scanner to create 3D visualizations is impractical. It's like sitting in your car to read a book. You can do it, but if you're sitting in the car, you may as well be driving. CT scanners are expensive pieces of equipment, and any process that hinders using the scanner to image patients is misappropriation of resources, unless no one is waiting to be scanned. Furthermore, a busy, crowded CT scan console is not the optimal location for interpreting imaging data. It is rarely possible to study the data in a meaningful way in this environment. The use of these tools is best left for emergency situations and for highly scripted visualizations that CT technologists create in association with specific clinical protocols, such as vertebral reformations.

- *3D workstations.* Most 3D workstations are stand-alone devices that offer a variety of the visualization tools discussed earlier. In general, the most advanced 3D processing tools are found on stand-alone workstations. They are invaluable for routine 3D image creation, particularly when 3D image creation and analysis can be localized to the site where the workstation is placed. Unlike PACS, however, 3D workstations do not typically function in a distributed manner throughout a radiology department or medical center. The workstations tend to be expensive and thus placing workstations at all locations where 3D interactivity is desired may be impractical. Recent developments from some vendors are focusing on interactivity and data sharing between workstations; however, it is too early to tell what their impact will be.

- *Distributed 3D systems.* These setups permit the simultaneous rendering of multiple data sets on a networked computer system consisting of a single 3D server and numerous client workstations. The server has a large amount of random-access memory (RAM) and hard drive space, as well as high-performance central and graphics processing units. The server is controlled by "thin" client workstations that are standard PCs running small applications that instruct the server and then display the renderings that the server generates. Although the thin-client workstation usually does not offer all the advanced tools that a dedicated 3D workstation provides, it has the advantage of being inexpensive and thus practical to locate anywhere in the department that has a fast network connection to the server. Pre-existing PCs may suffice for this purpose and thus, with the acquisition of a single server, an innumerable number of 3D clients can be set up on existing PCs, in convenient locations such as radiologists' offices, clinics, hospital wards, conference rooms, and operating rooms.

Conclusions

The latest advances in radiological imaging, in particular MDCT, have been accompanied by an explosion of data, requiring the implementation of fast and capacious computer systems for managing the information flow. Currently, patient preparation and actual CT scanning represent a small part of the total workflow, while data transfer, image reconstruction, 3D processing, interpretation, and archiving are time-consuming, expensive, and elaborate activities. Optimal data transfer is achieved with fast networks and powerful computers. Accurate image interpretation is no longer feasible by visual assessment, and requires sophisticated, dedicated software for 3D visualization and volumetric analysis. Finally, CT studies must be archived temporarily in capacious hard disks or in digital "offline" libraries for long-term storage. In order to fully benefit from the clinical advantages of MDCT, further developments in both hardware and software are necessary, and radiology departments must maintain adequate computing facilities as support to the increasing clinical workflow.

References

1. Rubin GD, Napel S, Leung A (1996) Volumetric analysis of volume data: achieving a paradigm shift. Radiology 200:312-317
2. Keller PJ, Drayer BP, Fram EK et al (1989) MR angiography with two-dimensional acquisition and three-dimensional display. Radiology 173:527-532
3. Napel S, Rubin GD, Jeffrey Jr (1993) RB. STS-MIP: A new reconstruction technique for CT of the chest. J Comput Assist Tomogr; 17:832-838.
4. Rubin GD (1996) Techniques of reconstruction. In: Rémy-Jardin M, Rémy J (eds) Spiral CT of the chest.

Springer, Berlin Heidelberg New York, pp 101-128

5. Zeman RK, Berman PM, Silverman PM, Davros WJ, Cooper C, Kladakis AO, Gomes MN (1995) Diagnosis of aortic dissection: value of helical CT with multiplanar reformation and three-dimensional rendering. AJR Am J Roentgenol 164:1375-1380

6. Cline HE, Lorensen WE, Souza SP et al (1991) 3D Surface rendered MR images of the brain and its vasculature. J Comput Assist Tomogr 15:344-351

7. Magnusson M, Lenz R, Danielsson PE (1991) Evaluation of methods for shaded surface display of CT volumes. Comput Med Imaging Graph 15:247-256

8. Rubin GD, Dake MD, Napel S et al (1994) Spiral CT of renal artery stenosis: comparison of three-dimensional rendering techniques. Radiology 190:181-189

9. Drebin RA, Carpenter L, Hanrahan P (1998) Volume rendering. Comput Graphics 22:65-74

10. Levoy M (1991) Methods for improving the efficiency and versatility of volume rendering. Prog Clin Biol Res 363:473-488

11. Rusinek H, Mourino MR, Firooznia H et al (1989) Volumetric rendering of MR images. Radiology 171:269-272

12. Fishman EK, Drebin B, Magid D et al (1987) Volumetric rendering techniques: applications for three-dimensional imaging of the hip. Radiology 163:737-738

13. Rubin GD, Beaulieu CF, Argiro V et al (1996) Perspective volume rendering of CT and MR images: applications for endoscopic imaging. Radiology 199:321-330

14. Johnson PT, Heath DG, Bliss DF et al (1996) Three-dimensional CT: real-time interactive volume rendering. AJR Am J Roentgenol 167:581-583

15. Kuszyk BS, Heath DG, Bliss DF et al (1996) Skeletal 3-D CT: advantages of volume rendering over surface rendering. Skeletal Radiol 25:207-214

16. Hara AK, Johnson CD, Reed JE et al (1996) Colorectal polyp detection with CT colography: two- versus three-dimensional techniques. Work in progress [see comments]. Radiology 200:49-54

17. Hara AK, Johnson CD, Reed JE et al (1996) Detection of colorectal polyps by computed tomographic colography: feasibility of a novel technique. Gastroenterology 110:284-290

18. Ferretti GR, Vining DJ, Knoplioch J et al (1996) Tracheobronchial tree: three-dimensional spiral CT with bronchoscopic perspective. J Comput Assist Tomogr 20:777-781

19. Vining DJ, Liu K, Choplin RH et al (1996) Virtual bronchoscopy. Relationships of virtual reality endobronchial simulations to actual bronchoscopic findings. Chest 109:549-553

20. Naidich DP, Grudrn JF, McGuinness G et al (1997) Volumetric (helical/spiral) CT (VCT) of the airways. J Thoracic Imaging 12:11-28

21. Kimura F, Shen Y, Date S et al (1996) Thoracic aortic aneurysm and aortic dissection: new endoscopic mode for three-dimensional CT display of aorta. Radiology 198:573-578

22. Vining DJ, Zagoria RJ, Liu K et al (1996) CT cystoscopy: an innovation in bladder imaging. AJR Am J Roentgenol 166:409-410

23. Sommer FG, Olcott EW, Ch'en IY et al (1997) Volume rendering of CT data: applications to the genitourinary tract. AJR Am J Roentgenol 168:1223-1226

IV.4

Late Adverse Events Following Administration of Iodinated Contrast Media: An Update

Alberto Spinazzi

Introduction

With the advent of multidetector-computed tomography (MDCT) technology, the number of patients undergoing contrast-enhanced CT studies has steadily grown in the last 6 years. In 2003, it was in the order of 18 million in the European Union and 24 million in the United States. Post-contrast adverse events, i.e., all those unintended and unfavorable signs, symptoms, or diseases temporally associated with the use of an iodinated contrast medium (CM), are a fact of life in radiology departments. Most adverse events occur within the first 60 min following the CM administration, with the greatest risk in the first 5 min. More delayed CM adverse events do occur, with some events recorded up to 7 days after CM administration, although a significant proportion of delayed adverse events are probably unrelated to CM administration. Among all types of delayed adverse events, only delayed hypersensitivity skin reactions are well-documented untoward side effects of CM. Besides delayed skin reactions, contrast-induced nephropathy (CIN) is also a serious, well-known, late complication of CM use. This chapter is aimed at summarizing the most recent literature on CIN and late skin reactions.

Contrast-Induced Nephropathy

Definition, Epidemiology, and Clinical Features

CIN is an acute decline in renal function after administration of an iodinated CM in the absence of an alternative cause [1, 2]. Development of CIN is defined by a transient increase in the concentration of serum creatinine (SCr) relative to baseline levels. The definition of the point at which a patient develops CIN varies from clinical study to clinical study. Definitions range from absolute (0.5–1.0 mg/dl) to relative (10%, 25%, 50%, or 100%) increases over baseline levels. In the vast majority of clinical trials, however, CIN has been defined as a relative rise in SCr $\geq$25%, or as an absolute increase of $\geq$0.5 mg/dl from baseline [3, 4]. Based on this definition, the overall incidence of CIN is estimated to be 0.6%–2.3% [5]. In patients with cardiovascular pathology undergoing angiography procedures, the incidence of CIN is higher and ranges from 3.3% to 14.5% [6, 7]. Chronic kidney disease, defined as SCr persistently >1.5 mg/dl or a calculated or estimated creatinine clearance (CrCl) <60 ml/min per 1.73 m^2, is the most-important factor for the development of CIN [1, 2, 6]. Other major risk factors for CIN include dehydration, diabetes mellitus, any condition associated with decreased effective circulating volume, and use of large CM doses [1, 2, 6] (Table 1).

The most common features of CIN are shown in Table 2. The rise in SCr usually occurs within 24–48 h of exposure to iodinated CM, with a return to baseline or near baseline within 7-10 days in most cases [3, 8]. Dialysis as a result of CIN is required in 0.3%–0.7% of patients undergoing angiography [6, 7]. Almost every patient who develops acute renal failure requiring dialysis shows a significant SCr rise at 24 h after the exposure to iodinated CM [9]. Patients who develop contrast-induced acute renal failure are at significantly higher risk of death, both in hospital and long term [6, 10-12]. The prognosis is particularly unfavorable in patients with pre-existing renal compromise [10, 11].

Table 1. Risk factors for contrast-induced nephropathy (CIN)

Established	Probable
• Dehydration	• Age >70 years
• Pre-existing renal failure	• Female gender
• Diabetes mellitus	• Concomitant use of loop diuretics
• Large contrast volume	• Concurrent administration of drugs that are directly nephrotoxic
• Repeat contrast in <48 h	or produce intra-renal vasoconstriction (cyclosporin,
• Class III/IV CHF	aminoglycosides, antineoplastic agents, amphotericin B,
• Multiple myeloma	dipyridamole, adenosine, etc.)

(*CHF* = congestive heart failure)

Table 2. Clinical features of contrast-induced nephropathy (CIN)

- SCr rise occurs within the first 24 h (80% of cases) or at 48–72 h (20% of cases), and peaks at 3–5 days
- Most common feature of CIN is a transient, self-resolving increase in SCr ("benign creatininopathy")
  - Nonoliguric
  - Urinalysis may reveal granular casts, tubular epithelial cells, and minimal proteinuria
  - SCr returns to baseline values within 7–10 days
- In a minority of cases, CIN leads to serious renal failure requiring either nephrology consultation or dialysis
  - Nearly all patients who progress to serious ARF have a rise in SCr within the first 24 h

(*SCr* = serum creatinine, *ARF* = acute renal failure)

CIN Following Intra-arterial Administration of CM in Patients with Renal Impairment

Literature Search Methodology. Several studies have evaluated the nephrotoxicity of nonionic monomers and dimers in patients with renal failure undergoing cardiac or peripheral angiography. A systematic and comprehensive on-line search was performed for publications printed from January 1991 to April 2004. The search included the following databases: EMBASE, MEDLINE, Biosis Previews, Derwent Drug File, Pascal, and SciSearch Cited Ref Sci. The following criteria were prospectively defined to select studies for inclusion in the review:

(1) English language.
(2) Publication in peer-reviewed journals.
(3) Either randomized, double-blind comparisons of iodinated contrast media or prospective, controlled studies of the safety and efficacy of pharmacological measures for the prevention of CIN (*N*-acetylcysteine or other drugs).
(4) The exact number or proportion of patients who had received a specific nonionic contrast agent (e.g., iodixanol, iohexol, iopamidol, etc.) was clearly reported.
(5) The exact number of patients who had received or not received any preventive measure other than hydration was clearly reported.
(6) Adequate hydration before and after the procedure.
(7) Study populations with mean baseline SCr levels between 1.5 and 2.5 mg/dl and/or mean baseline CrCl between 40 and 60 ml/min.
(8) Intra-arterial administration.
(9) Measurement of CIN as an absolute increase of ≥0.5 mg/dl or a relative increase of >25% in SCr over baseline at 48–72 h after the administration of the CM

Fourteen studies met the predefined selection criteria, 3 with iohexol (Omnipaque), 3 with iodixanol (Visipaque), 1 with iohexol and iodixanol, 4 with iopamidol (Iopamiro, Solutrast, Jopamiro, Niopam, Isovue), 1 with iomeprol (Iomeron), 1 with iopromide (Ultravist), and 1 with ioxilan (Oxilan). To eliminate the confounding effect of drug premedication and ensure consistency, only the data from patients who had received a nonionic contrast agent and no premedication have been reviewed, i.e., from the control arm of the studies conducted to evaluate the preventive efficacy of acetylcysteine or other drugs, or of the patients who had received a nonionic agent in the comparisons of contrast agents.

CIN Rates Following Intra-arterial Administration of Iohexol in Risk Patients. Rudnick et al. [13] conducted a double-blind, randomized study to compare the incidence of nephrotoxicity with diatrizoate and iohexol in 1,196 patients undergoing cardiac angiography. Patients were divided into four groups based on the presence of renal insufficiency and diabetes mellitus as follows: (a) neither renal insufficiency nor diabetes mellitus, (b) diabetes mellitus but no renal insufficiency, (c) renal insufficiency but no diabetes mellitus, and (d) renal insufficiency and diabetes mellitus present. A total of 250 patients had pre-existing renal failure in the iohexol-treated group, 102 were also diabetic. Mean baseline SCr values were 1.8±0.6 mg/dl in all patients with renal compromise and 2.0±0.6 mg/dl in those with renal failure and diabetes mellitus. CIN, defined as an increase in SCr of ≥0.5 mg/dl from baseline within 48–72 h of CM administration, occurred in 52 of 250 patients (20.8%). In patients with concomitant diabetes, the incidence of CIN was higher (34/102, 33.3%). Among the patients with renal failure that experienced CIN after the administration of iohexol, 9 also experienced unusually severe nephrotoxicity, and 5 of these patients (2%) ultimately required acute dialysis.

Durham et al. [14] conducted a double-blind study to assess the possible preventive effect of *N*-acetylcysteine in 81 angiography patients with SCr levels of at least 1.7 mg/dl. Patients were randomized into groups receiving prophylaxis for CIN with intravenous saline only (control group) versus intravenous saline plus *N*-acetylcysteine. All patients received iohexol, and CIN was defined as an increase in SCr of at least 0.5 mg/dl at 48 h. At the end of the study, 79 patients were available for analysis. The results showed that 24% of patients experienced CIN after iohexol (26% in the treatment group and 22% in the control arm). In diabetic subjects the results were even worse, with 42% of the acetylcysteine group and 28% of the control group experiencing CIN. In all, 5 of 79 (6.3%) patients experienced SCr increases of greater than 1.0 mg/dl, and 2 patients experienced SCr increases of over 2.0 mg/dl. For these patients (3% of the patient population) dialysis was required.

Hans et al. [15] prospectively studied 55 patients with chronic renal insufficiency who underwent abdominal arteriography and arteriography of the lower extremities. The patients were randomized into two groups, one (28 patients) that received dopamine and one (27 patients) that received an equal volume of saline and no premedication. All patients received iohexol, and CIN was defined as an increase in SCr of at least 0.5 mg/dl at 24-96 h after angiography. At 48-72 h after examination, 10 of the 27 patients (37%) in the iohexol-saline group experienced CIN.

In Aspelin's NEPHRIC study [16], all the study patients had diabetes mellitus and pre-existing renal failure (mean baseline SCr 1.6±0.5 mg/dl). A peak increase in SCr of ≥0.5 mg/dl was observed in 17 of 65 (26%) patients receiving iohexol. Six patients (9%) had clinical acute renal failure related to the use of iohexol and had to undergo hemodialysis. Three of these patients recovered, two died, one had persistent renal failure.

Figure 1 shows the incidence of CIN observed with Omnipaque. Overall, the incidence of CIN in patients with renal compromise enrolled in these studies was 21%-37% (mean 23.0%).

CIN Rates Following Intra-arterial Administration of iodixanol in Risk Patients. The RAPPID study by Baker [17] evaluated the efficacy of intravenous acetylcysteine in the prevention of the nephrotoxic effects of iodixanol in patients with moderate renal failure (baseline SCr levels 1.75±0.41 mg/dl, baseline CrCl 44±18 ml/min). The patients in the RAPPID study who were not randomized to receive the antioxidant had intravenous hydration for 12 h before receiving iodixanol. There were two groups, one receiving acetylcysteine premedication and one receiving only saline. The incidence

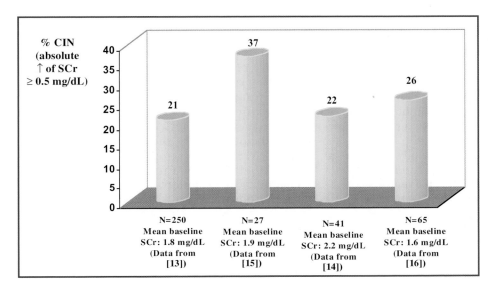

Fig. 1. Incidence of contrast-induced nephropathy following administration of low-osmolar monomer iohexol in patients with renal impairment (Data from [13-16])

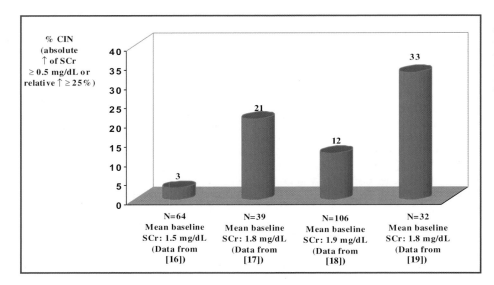

Fig. 2. Incidence of contrast-induced nephropathy following administration of the iso-osmolar dimer iodixanol in patients with renal impairment. (Data from [16-19])

of CIN (SCr increases of 25%) was 21% (8/39 patients) following iodixanol and no premedication with acetylcysteine.

Boccalandro et al. [18] published a randomized, double-blind trial comparing the renal tolerability of iodixanol-enhanced interventional cardiac angiographic procedures with or without pretreatment with oral acetylcysteine in 181 patients with moderate chronic renal insufficiency. All patients were hydrated for 12 h prior to the procedure. Baseline SCr in the study group receiving iodixanol and no premedication was 1.9 mg/dl. Baseline CrCl was 50±29 ml/min. The mean increase in SCr following iodixanol and hydration was 0.19±0.4. The incidence of CIN (SCr increase >0.5 mg/dl at 48 h after CM administration) was 12% (13/106).

Recently, Stone et al. [19] conducted a randomized, double-blind, placebo-controlled study of 315 patients with moderate to severe renal failure to examine the efficacy of fenoldopam mesylate, a specific agonist of the dopamine-1 receptor, in preventing CIN after invasive cardiovascular procedures. Iodixanol was used in 10% of patients. CIN (SCr increase of ≥0.5 mg/dl) occurred in 33.3% of patients who received the iso-osmolar iodixanol, compared with 25.3% of those who received low-osmolar agents.

The results of the NEPHRIC study [16] showed that iodixanol induced a mean increase in SCr of 0.13 mg/dl. Peak increases of >0.5 mg/dl were observed in 3% of patients (2/64 patients). There were no patients with a peak increase >1.0 mg/dl.

Figure 2 shows the incidence of CIN with Visipaque. Overall, the incidence of CIN in patients with renal compromise enrolled in these studies was 3%-33% (mean 14%).

CIN Rates Following Intra-arterial Administration of Iopamidol in Risk Patients. Taliercio et al. [20] compared the nephrotoxicity of diatrizoate and iopamidol. In this randomized, double-blind clinical trial, 307 patients with renal impairment undergoing cardiac angiography were enrolled. Renal impairment was defined as SCr ≥1.5 mg/dl at recruitment; the mean baseline SCr for the entire population was 2.02 mg/dl. At the 24-h evaluation, mean SCr levels were significantly increased in the diatrizoate group compared with the iopamidol group. The mean maximal rise in SCr was significantly higher in the diatrizoate group compared with the iopamidol group. The maximal SCr rise was >0.5 mg/dl in 8% of iopamidol patients versus 19% of diatrizoate patients. A multivariate analysis of the effects of contrast agent, diabetes mellitus requiring insulin, and the presence of severe renal insufficiency (i.e., baseline SCr >3 mg/dl) revealed that a greater maximal change in SCr was independently related to the use of diatrizoate, the presence of diabetes mellitus requiring insulin, and the presence of severe renal insufficiency. These results indicate that iopamidol was less nephrotoxic than diatrizoate in patients with renal insufficiency.

Coincident with the publication of the NEPHRIC study, Kay et al. [21] published a randomized, double-blind trial comparing the renal tolerability of iopamidol-enhanced diagnostic or interventional cardiac angiographic procedures with or without pretreatment with oral acetylcysteine in 200 patients with moderate chronic renal insufficiency (CrCl <60 ml/min). Patients had intravenous hydration for 12 h before receiving iopamidol and for 6 h after. Mean baseline SCr lev-

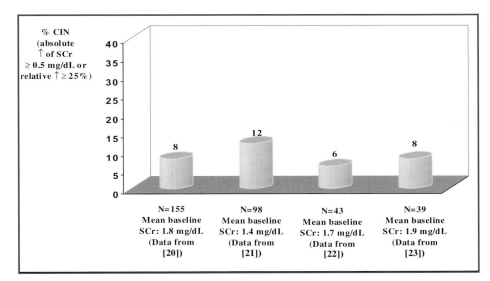

Fig. 3. Incidence of contrast-induced nephropathy following administration of the low-osmolar monomer iopamidol in patients with renal impairment. (Data from [20-23])

els were 1.36 mg/dl and mean baseline CrCl was 45.0 (range 12.7–59.8) ml/min in the group receiving iopamidol alone. The incidence of CIN (SCr increase of 25%) was 12% without premedication with acetylcysteine and 4% following premedication with the antioxidant. No patient developed clinical acute renal failure following iopamidol. Without any premedication, SCr levels showed a decrease 24 h after the iopamidol-enhanced cardiac angiography procedure, and very modest increases (mean SCr increase 0.02 mg/dl) 2 and 7 days after CM administration. An increase in CrCl was even observed in patients receiving iopamidol without premedication, in the whole group as well as in subgroups with chronic renal failure and diabetes, and with reduced (30%–50%) left ventricular ejection fraction. This means that, if any, the deterioration of the renal function of the study patients was minimal or negligible, even in the presence of well-known risk factors for CIN.

Oldemeyer et al. [22] conducted another randomized, double-blind, placebo-controlled trial to assess the preventive effect of oral acetylcysteine in 96 patients with moderate chronic renal failure undergoing elective coronary angiography with iopamidol. All patients received half-isotonic (0.45%) saline at 1 ml/kg per hour intravenously for 12 h before and 12 h after angiography. The primary study endpoint was the development of CIN, defined as an absolute increase in SCr of $\geq$0.5 mg/dl from baseline or a relative increase of $\geq$25% at 24 and 48 h after the procedure. CIN occurred in 8.2% (4/49) of patients taking acetylcysteine and 6.4% (3/47) of patients taking placebo. In patients with superimposed diabetes mellitus, the incidence of CIN was 15% (3/20) in acetylcysteine-treated patients and 8.7% (2/23) in placebo-treated patients. No patient developed acute renal failure or required dialysis.

Very recently, Goldenberg et al. [23] published the results of another placebo-controlled, double-blind trial assessing the preventive efficacy of oral acetylcysteine in patients with chronic renal failure (mean baseline SCr 1.9±0.3 mg/dl) receiving iopamidol. All patients received half-isotonic (0.45%) saline at 1 ml/kg per hour intravenously for 12 h before and 12 h after coronary angiography. The primary study endpoint was the development of CIN, defined as an absolute increase in SCr of $\geq$0.5 mg/dl from baseline at 48 h after coronary angiography. CIN occurred in 10% (4/41) of patients in the acetylcysteine group and in 8% (3/39) of patients in the placebo group.

Figure 3 shows the incidence of CIN in studies with Isovue. Overall, the incidence of CIN in patients with renal compromise enrolled in these studies was 8%–12% (mean 9%).

CIN Rates Following Intra-arterial Administration of Other Nonionic Monomers. Huber et al. [24] investigated whether the adenosine antagonist theophylline could prevent or reduce CIN in patients with chronic renal insufficiency (SCr level at baseline 2.07±0.94 mg/dl). Fifty patients were randomized to receive iomeprol and placebo and 50 patients were randomized to receive 200 mg theophylline intravenously 30 min before angiography with iomeprol. High doses of CM were used for diagnostic or interventional procedures (always >150 ml, 250–349 ml in 15 patients, >350 ml in 10 patients, mean±SD 216.6±95.0 ml in the iomeprol-placebo group, 196.5±84.1 ml in the iomeprol-theophylline group). The majority of patients (86% in the iomeprol-placebo group, 88% in the iomeprol-theophylline group) received concomitant nephrotoxic medications (aminoglycoside, vancomycin, nonsteroidal anti-inflammatory drugs, amphotericin B, and/or nephrotoxic chemotherapy). Several patients also suffered from diabetes mellitus (40% in the iomeprol-placebo group, 28% in the iomeprol-theophylline group). The overall incidence of CIN (SCr increase of ≥0.5 mg/dl) was 10% (16% in the placebo group, 4% in the theophylline group). The incidence of CIN in the subset of patients with renal failure and diabetes was 10% in the iomeprol-placebo group. None of the patients developed acute renal failure.

Briguori et al. [25] conducted a placebo-controlled study in 183 consecutive patients with renal impairment to evaluate the prophylactic effect of intravenous acetylcysteine. The contrast agent used was iopromide in all patients. Patients in the placebo group had a baseline SCr level of 1.5±0.4 mg/dl. CIN was defined as an increase of ≥25% over baseline levels in the 48 h following the angiographic procedure. The incidence of CIN in the subset of patients treated with placebo (saline) was 11% (10/91 patients).

Diaz-Sandoval et al. [26] used the nonionic monomer ioxilan in 54 patients with chronic renal failure; 25 patients received oral acetylcysteine, 29 a placebo (saline). Mean baseline SCr was 1.66±0.05 mg/dl in the pretreated group and 1.56±0.04 in the ioxilan-placebo group. The incidence of CIN (SCr increase of ≥25% over baseline) in the placebo group was 45%.

CIN Following Intravenous administration

There are fewer studies assessing the renal safety of iodinated agents following their intravenous administration. Two studies compared two different nonionic monomers with iodixanol. The first double-blind comparison of the effects of the iso-osmolar iodixanol and the low-osmolar iopromide on renal function in 64 patients with mild-to-moderate renal insufficiency was conducted by Carraro et al. [27] Patients with SCr values between 1.5 and 3.0 mg/dl underwent excretory urography with one of the two randomly assigned CM. Renal function was assessed before and 1, 6, 24, and 48 h, and 7 days after urography. Parameters included SCr, as well as urinary tubular enzymes (alanylaminopeptidase and N-acetyl-β-glucosaminidase), α_1-microglobulin, and albumin. Baseline characteristics between the two groups were similar. SCr levels decreased during the observation period in both groups, but no statistical difference between treatments was noted. One nondiabetic patient in the Visipaque group devel-

oped CIN (SCr increasing from 2.5 to 5.4 mg/dl in 24 h, returning to baseline by the 48-h evaluation). Overall, neither alanylaminopeptidase nor N-acetyl-β-glucosaminidase changed significantly in either treatment group, although 1 patient in the Visipaque group had an increase in N-acetyl-β-glucosaminidase of almost 700 mU/mg urinary creatinine from baseline to 24 h. Levels of α_1-microglobulin and albumin did not change during the observation period, nor did blood pressure or heart rate.

A more-recent study compared the isotonic dimer iodixanol with the low-osmolar, nonionic monomer iobitridol in 50 patients undergoing cranial or body CT procedures [28]. Both groups received similar volumes of CM (113.3 ml of iobitridol, 112.7 ml of iodixanol) and had similar baseline values of SCr (2.7 mg/dl, i.e., 242.0 μmol/l in the iobitridol group, 2.6 mg/dl, i.e., 229.7 μmol/l in the iodixanol group) and CrCl (28.7 ml/min vs. 27.5 ml/min). No differences were observed between the two agents. The SCr increase was ≥0.5 mg/dl, i.e., 44 μmol/l, in 17% of patients with both agents, while a decrease of CrCl of ≥25% was observed in 12.5% of patients with both agents. In both studies, the renal safety of the nonionic dimeric agent was identical to that of the nonionic monomeric agents.

A recently published study by Haight et al. [29], partially sponsored by the National Cancer Institute, evaluated the renal tolerability of iopamidol in pediatric patients (median age 8.1 years) undergoing CT following bone marrow transplantation. These patients received several immunosuppressive and antimicrobial drugs that are quite nephrotoxic (cyclosporin A, methotrexate, cytarabine, aminoglycosides, amphotericin B, acyclovir, etc.). CT is the examination of choice for the detection of foci of infection and other complications in these patients. The study assessed the possible potentiation of nephrotoxicity following relatively high doses (2–3 ml/kg) of contrast agents. In this study, iopamidol showed no or negligible effects on the kidney function of those pediatric patients that were definitely at higher than usual risk for the development of acute renal failure following CM administration.

Steps for Prevention

The most effective strategy for minimizing the risk for CIN is careful patient assessment. When iodinated contrast-enhanced images are deemed necessary, a detailed medical history and physical examination should be performed. Identification of the co-morbid risk factors allows the physician to reduce the risk of CIN by proactively addressing these potential problems (Table 3). However,

Table 3. Nonpharmacological steps for prevention of CIN

1. Identify co-morbid risk factors
Look for:
• Age over 70 years
• Dehydration
• SCr >1.5 mg/dl (or, better, calculated creatinine clearance <60 ml/min), particularly as a result of diabetic nephropathy
• Congestive heart failure
• Concurrent administration of drugs that are directly nephrotoxic or produce intra-renal vasoconstriction (cyclosporin, aminoglycosides, antineoplastic agents, amphotericin B, dipyridamole, adenosine, etc.)
2. Nonpharmacological prophylactic measures
• Consider alternative imaging modalities that do not require the administration of iodinated CM
• Stop administration of nephrotoxic drugs for 24 h before and after the contrast-enhanced examination
• Stop administration of diuretics (especially loop diuretics)
• Stop administration of metformin for 48 h after CM administration
• Make sure the patient is well hydrated
• Limit the dose of CM
• Do not perform multiple imaging studies with iodinated contrast agents in a short period of time (keep an interval ≥72 h between contrast examinations)
• Use low- or iso-osmolar CM

Table 4. Steps for prevention of CIN: hydration

1. Patients should be properly hydrated before and after CM administration
2. Intravenous (IV) hydration reported to more effective than unrestricted oral fluids [30]
3. Isotonic (0.9% NaCl) IV hydration reported to be more effective than half-isotonic (0.45% NaCl) IV hydration [31]
• Maximum benefit of isotonic IV hydration for women, diabetics, patients receiving >250 ml CM
4. IV hydration with sodium bicarbonate reported to more effective than IV hydration with 0.9% NaCl [32]

many high-risk patients are not identified prior to undergoing contrast radiography studies. One survey found that only about 20% of practices in the United States routinely obtain SCr levels before CM administration [30]. No studies have evaluated the frequency with which physicians hydrate their patients prior to contrast studies. Prophylactic hydration with saline can correct the very important risk factor of dehydration. Also, saline hydration may help minimize the direct toxicity of the contrast agent, by reducing its intratubular concentration and retention. Trivedi et al. [31] reported that intravenous hydration was more effective than unrestricted oral fluids. Mueller et al. [32] reported that intravenous hydration with isotonic (0.9% sodium chloride) saline is more effective at preventing CIN than hydration with half-isotonic (0.45% sodium chloride) saline. Recently, Merten et al. [33] randomized 119 patients to receive 0.9% solutions of either sodium bicarbonate or sodium chloride intravenously as a 3 ml/kg bolus per hour for 1 h prior to intra-arterial administration of a low-osmolar contrast agent, iopamidol. For 6 h after the contrast-enhanced procedure, all the study patients received an infusion of 0.9% sodium bicarbonate or 0.9% sodium chloride solutions at 1 ml/kg per hour. CIN, defined as an increase in SCr of 25% or more within 2 days of the angiographic procedure, occurred in 1.7% of the patients who received sodium bicarbonate and in 13.6% of the patients receiving sodium chloride (Table 4).

Another standard recommendation for reducing the potential for CIN is to use the lowest dose of CM possible, particularly in patients with reduced renal function. Several prophylactic drug treatments have been proposed, although an effective treatment to prevent CIN remains to be established.

Delayed Adverse Events Following Iodinated Contrast Agents

Definition and Clinical Features

A delayed adverse event (DAE) can be defined as an event occurring more than 1 h after the administration of an iodinated contrast agent. A temporal range of 1 h to 7 days has been suggested [34, 35]. Since DAEs usually occur after the patient has left the radiology department or the catheter laboratory, their relationship to the contrast-enhanced procedure is not easily recognized [35-37].

In DAEs, the symptoms that are more commonly reported are headache, dizziness, itching, nausea, vomiting, diarrhea, and skin reactions [34-37]. A significant proportion of DAEs is probably unrelated to CM administration. A study conducted to compare the incidence of DAEs following unenhanced and contrast-enhanced CT showed that DAEs occurred in 293 of 2,370 patients (12.4%) who received a nonionic monomeric CM and in 93 of 907 patients (10.3%) who did not receive any CM [38]. Among all types of DAEs, only delayed hypersensitivity skin reactions are well-documented untoward side effects of CM [36, 37]. The majority of the skin reactions are of the following types: urticaria, morbilliform/maculopapular eruptions, erythema multiform eruptions, and other nonspecific rashes [35, 37, 39-41]. Most of the skin reactions are usually not serious and mild or moderate in severity, i.e., they may cause discomfort and require specific treatment (steroids, antihistamines, topical emollients), but are rarely life threatening or require hospitalization [35-37, 39-41], and usually do not cause death or permanent disability. Depending on their localization, these delayed skin reactions may be more or less disturbing, the most troublesome being those confined to the palms, soles of the feet, or face [39].

Pathogenesis

Some suggest that DAEs are mediated by a type IV hypersensitivity reaction [34, 36, 40, 41], i.e., that they are T-cell mediated and involve antigen-specific T-lymphocytes, which respond specifically to an antigen by the release of lymphokines. This assumption is based on the described clinical history, skin test results, results from provocation testing, and description of the histological findings after skin and provocation testing [36, 40, 41]. If delayed hypersensitivity causes a DAE, the time frame for its onset is 48–72 h after dose administration.

Available skin test results indicate that the skin eruptions are caused by the iodinated contrast agent and not by the excipients [40, 41]. It has been shown that iodinated CM form molecular agglomerates that are larger and more stable the lower the osmolality and the higher the viscosity of the solution [42]. Therefore, the largest molecular agglomerates have been observed with the isotonic and highly viscous iodixanol solutions, the second largest with the other nonionic dimer iotrolan. The molecular aggregates detected in iodixanol and iotrolan solutions were much larger than those formed by the nonionic monomer iopamidol (14.0 nm and 11.8 nm vs. 4.0 nm, respectively) [42]. After intravascular injection, these agglomerates persist for some seconds or minutes in spite of the rapid dilution. During this period they may enter cells and stimulate them to mediate delayed hypersensitivity irrespective of the amount of contrast material that has already been excreted at the time of the reaction. The isotonic dimers iodixanol and iotrolan have been found to differ from nonionic monomers with respect to their retention (dwell time) in tissues, including skin, where they reach concentrations that are 2–3 times higher than those of monomers [42]. This difference between isotonic dimers and low-osmolar monomers may explain the higher frequency of late skin reactions following iotrolan and iodixanol in clinical trials [39, 43].

Some skin reactions (especially urticaria) may occur 1–24 h after dose administration. Direct release of mediators or direct complement activation, not a type IV hypersensitivity reaction, is probably involved in the genesis of earlier skin reactions 1–24 h after dose administration.

Frequency of Delayed Skin Reactions

The frequency of late skin reactions may vary according to the methodology used to collect the data (questionnaires, patient interviews in person, phone interviews), as well as according to the start points and duration of follow-up.

When contrast-enhanced CT is compared with unenhanced CT, the overall incidence of late skin reactions is 7.9%–11.6% with plain CT and 8.4%-14.9% following nonionic monomers [34, 38, 44]. In these studies, the difference in incidence between plain and contrast-enhanced CT ranged between 0.5% and 3.3%. Only skin reactions occurred more frequently following contrast, and their onset was usually between 1 and 3 days following the procedure.

Delayed skin reactions occur with higher incidence in patients with a history of adverse reactions to CM, a history of allergy, or with a SCr level of ≥2.0 mg/dl [45]. In a prospective survey of 15,890 patients undergoing CT examinations, 331 patients (2.1%) reported skin reactions; among

Table 5. Risk factors for delayed hypersensitivity reactions

- History of adverse reactions to CM
- History of allergy
- Chronic renal failure
- Season (spring/early summer)
- Previous or concurrent immunotherapy with interleukin-2
- Intravascular use of nonionic dimers

these 331 patients, 41 patients (12.4%) consulted a dermatologist [45]. A seasonal variation has been reported, with a peak incidence in late spring and early summer [46]. Although suggested, it is not clear whether females are more likely to develop DAEs than males [37]. It is well documented that delayed skin reactions are 2-4 times more frequent in patients who have received interleukin-2 immunotherapy [47-50].

No difference in DAE incidence has been observed between ionic and nonionic monomers [51-53], and among nonionic monomers [37, 52]. Significant differences have been found between the nonionic monomer iopamidol and the ionic dimer ioxaglate in the incidence of urticaria in the first 24 h after dose administration [39]. Delayed skin reactions are significantly more frequent with the isotonic dimers than with nonionic monomers [39, 43, 45]. A higher percentage of more severe skin reactions was observed when a nonionic dimer was used [45]. In another study, the frequency of skin reactions with a nonionic dimer was similar to that with a nonionic monomer, but specific treatment with steroids or antihistamines was more frequent with the isotonic dimer. Table 5 lists the established risk factors for late-onset, hypersensitivity skin reactions.

Conclusions

CIN and delayed hypersensitivity skin reactions are well known, relatively frequent, late complications of contrast-enhanced procedures. Risk factors for CIN and delayed skin reactions can be identified and corrected.

Nonpharmacological prophylactic measures can significantly reduce the incidence of CIN. High-risk patients for CIN should be properly identified and receive prior hydration and low-osmolar or iso-osmolar iodinated contrast. The risk of CIN with nonionic dimeric agents appears to be as low as with their nonionic monomeric counterparts in patients with pre-existing renal compromise. We reviewed the results of 14 prospective, controlled studies with similar design and endpoints. The acute deterioration of renal function varied across the reviewed studies and the contrast agents used. A higher incidence of CIN was observed after iohexol, while the risk of CIN with the nonionic dimer iodixanol appeared to be as low as that with the nonionic monomers iopamidol, iomeprol, iobitridol, and iopromide in patients with pre-existing renal compromise. The incidence of iodixanol-induced nephropathy was very low (3%) in the NEPHRIC study only [16]; other studies [17-19, 28] showed a higher incidence of CIN with this agent in angiography and CT (12%-33%). It is important to mention that serious complications may follow the administration of any iodinated contrast agent available on the market. A recent publication from the Royal London Hospital [54] reported cases of contrast nephropathy from a prospective survey of 267 patients. Of these patients, 46% had pre-existing renal impairment. The two contrast agents tested in the NEPHRIC study were the low-osmolar iohexol and the isotonic dimer iodixanol. CIN occurred after 15 procedures. There were 9 patients that died and 6 that recovered. Three deaths occurred directly as a result of CIN. One fatality occurred following the injection of iohexol and two fatalities occurred following injection of iodixanol for angiography.

Risk factors for delayed skin reactions are history of adverse reactions to contrast media, history of allergy, pre-existing renal impairment and immunotherapy with interleukin-2. Late skin reactions seem to be more frequent in spring/early summer. The majority of the delayed skin reactions are mild in intensity and self-resolving. However, they may be more severe, discomforting, and require specific treatment. The use of the isotonic nonionic dimers is associated with a higher frequency of delayed hypersensitivity reactions. Patients and treating physicians should be informed about the possibility of delayed skin reactions following a contrast-enhanced procedure.

References

1. Morcos SK, Thomsen HS, Webb JAW and members of the contrast media safety committee of the European Society of Urogenital Radiology (ESUR) (1999) Contrast media induced nephrotoxicity: A consensus report. Eur Radiol 9:1602-1613

2. Thomsen HS, Morcos SK (2003) Contrast media and the kidney: European Society of Urogenital Radiology (ESUR) Guidelines. Br J Radiol 76:513-518

3. McCullough PA, Sandberg KA (2003) Epidemiology of contrast-induced nephropathy. Rev Cardiovasc Med 4 [Suppl 5]:S3-S9

4. Thomsen HS (2003) Guidelines for contrast media from the European Society of Urogenital Radiology. AJR Am J Roentgenol 181:1463-1471

5. Lasser EC, Lyon SG, Barry CC (1997) Report on contrast media reactions: analysis of data from reports to the US Food and Drug Administration. Radiology 203:605-610

6. McCullough PA, Wolyn R, Racher LL et al (1997) Acute renal failure after coronary intervention: incidence, risk factors and relationship to mortality. Am J Med 103:368-375

7. Rihal CS, Textor SC, Grill DE et al (2002) Incidence and prognostic importance of acute renal failure after percutaneous coronary intervention. Circulation 105:2259-2264

8. Murphy SW, Barrett BJ, Parfrey PS (2000) Contrast nephropathy. J Am Soc Nephrol 11:177-182

9. Gutierrez N, Diaz A, Timmis GC et al (2002) Determinants of serum creatinine trajectory in acute contrast nephropathy. J Interv Cardiol 15:349-354

10. Levy EM, Viscoli CM, Horwitz RI (1996) The effect of acute renal failure on mortality. A cohort analysis. JAMA 275:1489-1494

11. Gruberg I, Mintz GS, Mehran R et al (2000) The prognostic implications of further renal function deterioration within 48 hours of intervention in patients with pre-existent chronic renal insufficiency. J Am Coll Cardiol 36:1542-1548

12. Best PJ, Lennon R, Ting HH et al (2002) The impact of renal insufficiency on clinical outcomes in patients undergoing percutaneous coronary interventions. J Am Coll Cardiol 39:1113-1119

13. Rudnick MR, Goldfarb S, Wexler L et al (1995) Nephrotoxicity of ionic and nonionic contrast media in 1196 patients: a randomized trial. Kidney Int 47:254-261

14. Durham JD, Caputo C, Dokko J et al (2002) A randomized controlled trial of N-acetyslcysteine to prevent contrast nephropathy in cardiac angiography. Kidney Int 62:2202-2207

15. Hans S, Hans BA, Dhillon R et al (1998) Effect of dopamine on renal function after arteriography in patients with pre-existing renal insufficiency. Am Surg 64:432-436

16. Aspelin P, Aubry P, Fransson SG et al (2003) Nephrotoxic effects in high-risk patients undergoing angiography. N Engl J Med 348:491-499

17. Baker CSR, Wragg A, Kumar S et al (2003) A rapid protocol for the prevention of contrast-induced renal dysfunction: the RAPPID study. J Am Coll Cardiol 41:2114-2118

18. Boccalandro F, Amhad M, Smalling RW, Sdringola S (2003) Oral acetylcysteine does not protect renal function from moderate to high doses of intravenous radiographic contrast. Cathet Cardiovasc Interv 58:336-341

19. Stone G, McCullough PA, Tumlin JA et al (2003) Fenoldopam mesylate for the prevention of contrast-induced nephropathy. A randomized controlled trial. JAMA 290:2284-2291

20. Taliercio CP, Vlietstra RE, Ilstrup DM et al (1991) A randomized comparison of nephrotoxicity of iopamidol and diatrizoate in high risk patients undergoing cardiac angiography. J Am Coll Cardiol 17:384-390

21. Kay J, Chow WH, Chan TM et al (2003) Acetylcysteine for prevention of acute deterioration of renal function following elective coronary angiography and intervention. JAMA 289:553-558

22. Oldemeyer JB, Biddle WP, Wurdeman RL et al (2003) Acetylcysteine in the prevention of contrast-induced nephropathy after coronary angiography. Am Heart J 146:e23

23. Goldenberg I, Shechter M, Matezky S et al (2004) Oral acetylcysteine as an adjunct to saline hydration for the prevention of contrast-induced nephropathy following coronary angiography. Eur Heart J 25:212-217

24. Huber W, Ilgmann K, Page M et al (2002) Effect of theophylline on contrast material-induced nephropathy in patients with chronic renal insufficiency: Controlled, randomized, double-blinded study. Radiology 223:772-779

25. Briguori C, Manganelli F, Scarpato P et al (2002) Acetylcysteine and contrast agent-associated nephrotoxicity. J Am Coll Cardiol 40:298-303

26. Diaz-Sandoval LJ, Kosowsky BD, Losordo DW (2002) Acetylcysteine to prevent angiography-related renal tissue injury (the APART trial). Am J Cardiol 89:356-358

27. Carraro M, Matalan F, Antonione P et al (1998) Effects of a dimeric vs a monomeric nonionic contrast medium on renal function in patients with mild to moderate renal insufficiency: a double-blind, randomized clinical trial. Eur Radiol 8:144-147

28. Kolehmainen H, Soiva M (2003) Comparison of Xenetix 300 and Visipaque 320 in patients with renal failure. Eur Radiol 13:B32-B33

29. Haight AE, Kaste SC, Goloubeva OG et al (2003) Nephrotoxocity of iopamidol in pediatric, adolescent, and young adult patients who have undergone allogeneic bone marrow transplantation. Radiology 226:399-404

30. Lee JK, Warshauer DM, Bush WH Jr et al (1995) Determination of serum creatinine level before intravenous administration of iodinated contrast medium. A survey. Invest Radiol 30:700-705

31. Trivedi HS, Moore H, Nasr S et al (2003) A randomized prospective trial to assess the role of saline hydration on the development of contrast nephropathy. Nephron Clin Pract 93:C29-C34

32. Mueller C, Buerkle G, Buettner HJ et al (2002) Prevention of contrast media-associated nephropathy. Randomized comparison of 2 hydration regimens in 1620 patients undergoing coronary angioplasty. Arch Intern Med 162:329-336

33. Merten GJ, Burgess WP, Gray LV et al (2004) Prevention of contrast-induced nephropathy with sodium bicarbonate. A randomized controlled trial. JAMA 291:2328-2334

34. Yasuda R, Munechika H (1998) Delayed adverse reactions to nonionic monomeric contrast-enhanced media. Invest Radiol 33:1-5

35. Christiansen C, Pichler WJ, Skotland T (2000) Delayed allergy-like reactions to X-ray contrast media: mechanistic considerations. Eur Radiol 10:1965-1975

36. Yoshikawa H (1992) Late adverse reactions to non-ionic contrast media. Radiology 183:737-740
37. Webb JAW, Stacul F, Thomsen HS et al (2003) Members Of The Contrast Media Safety Committee Of The European Society Of Urogenital Radiology, Late adverse reactions to intravascular iodinated contrast media. Eur Radiol 13:181-184
38. Munechika H (1996) Delayed reaction of monomeric contrast media: comparison of plain and enhanced computed tomography. Eur Radiol 6:S16
39. Sutton AGC, Finn P, Grech ED et al (2001) Early and late reactions after the use of iopamidol 340, ioxaglate 32 and iodixanol 320 in cardiac catheterization. Am Heart J 141:677-683
40. Sanchez-Perez J, F-Villalta MG, Ruiz SA et al (2003) Delayed hypersensitivity reaction to the non-ionic X-ray contrast medium Visipaque (iodixanol). Contact Dermatitis 48:167
41. Vernassiere C, Trechot P, Commun N et al (2004) Low negative predictive value of skin tests in investigating delayed reactions to radio-contrast media. Contact Dermatitis 50:359-366
42. Speck U, Bohle F, Krause W et al (1998) Delayed hypersensitivity to X-ray CM: possible mechanisms and models. Acad Radiol 5 [Suppl 1]:S162-S165
43. Sutton AGC, Finn P, Campbell PG et al (2003) Early and late reactions following the use of iopamidol 340, iomeprol 350 and iodixanol 320 in cardiac catheterization. J Invas Cardiol 15:133-138
44. Ueda S, Mori H, Matsumoto S et al (2001) True delayed adverse reactions to non-ionic contrast media: a cohort analytic study. Eur Radiol 11 [Suppl 1]:377
45. Hoyosa T, Yamaguchi K, Akutsu T et al (2000) Delayed adverse reactions to iodinated contrast media and their risk factors. Radiat Med 18:39-45
46. Mikkonen R, Vehmas T, Granlund H et al (2000) Seasonal variation in the occurrence of late adverse skin reactions to iodine-based contrast media. Acta Radiol 41:390
47. Choyke PL, Miller DL, Lotze MT et al (1992) Delayed skin reactions to contrast media after interleukin2 immunotherapy. Radiology 183:111-114
48. Oldham RK, Brogley J, Braud E (1990) Contrast medium "recalls" interleukin-2 toxicity. J Clin Oncol 8:942-943
49. Shulman KL, Thompson JA, Benyunes MC et al (1993) Adverse reaction to intravenous contrast media in patients treated with interleukin-2. J Immunother 13:208-212
50. Zukiwski AA, David CL Coan J et al (1990) Increased incidence of hypersensitivity to iodine-containing radiographic contrast media after interleukin-2 administration. Cancer 65:1521-1524
51. Panto PN, Davies P (1986) Delayed reactions to urographic contrast media. Br J Radiol 59:41-44
52. Pedersen SH, Svaland MG, Reiss AL et al (1998) Late allergy-like reactions following vascular administration of radiography contrast media. Acta Radiol 39:344-348
53. McCullough M, Davies P, Richardson R (1989) A large trial of intravenous Conray 325 and Niopam 300 to assess immediate and delayed reactions. Br J Radiol 62:260-265
54. Srodon P, Matson M, Ham R (2003) Contrast nephropathy in lower limb angiography. Ann R Coll Surg Engl 85:177-191